AN ILLUSTRATED HISTORY OF THE
ROYAL NORTHERN HOSPITAL
1856–1992

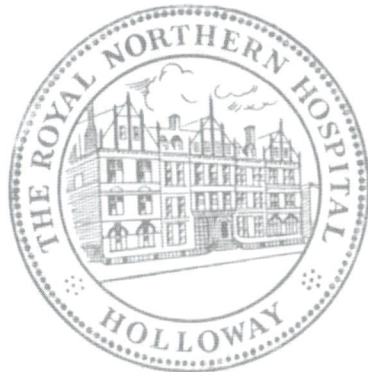

DR ALBERT RINSLER
MRCGP DHMSA

Published by Dr Albert Rinsler
© Dr Albert Rinsler 2007

ISBN 978-0-9555202-0-4

Designed by Angela Scott, UCL Media Resources

Printed by Stephen Austin & Sons Limited,
Caxton Hill, Hertford SG13 7LU

Distributed by the Press Office,
Jenner Building, Whittington Hospital,
Magdala Avenue, London N19 5NF
Telephone: **020 7288 5983**
E-mail: **communications@whittington.nhs.uk**

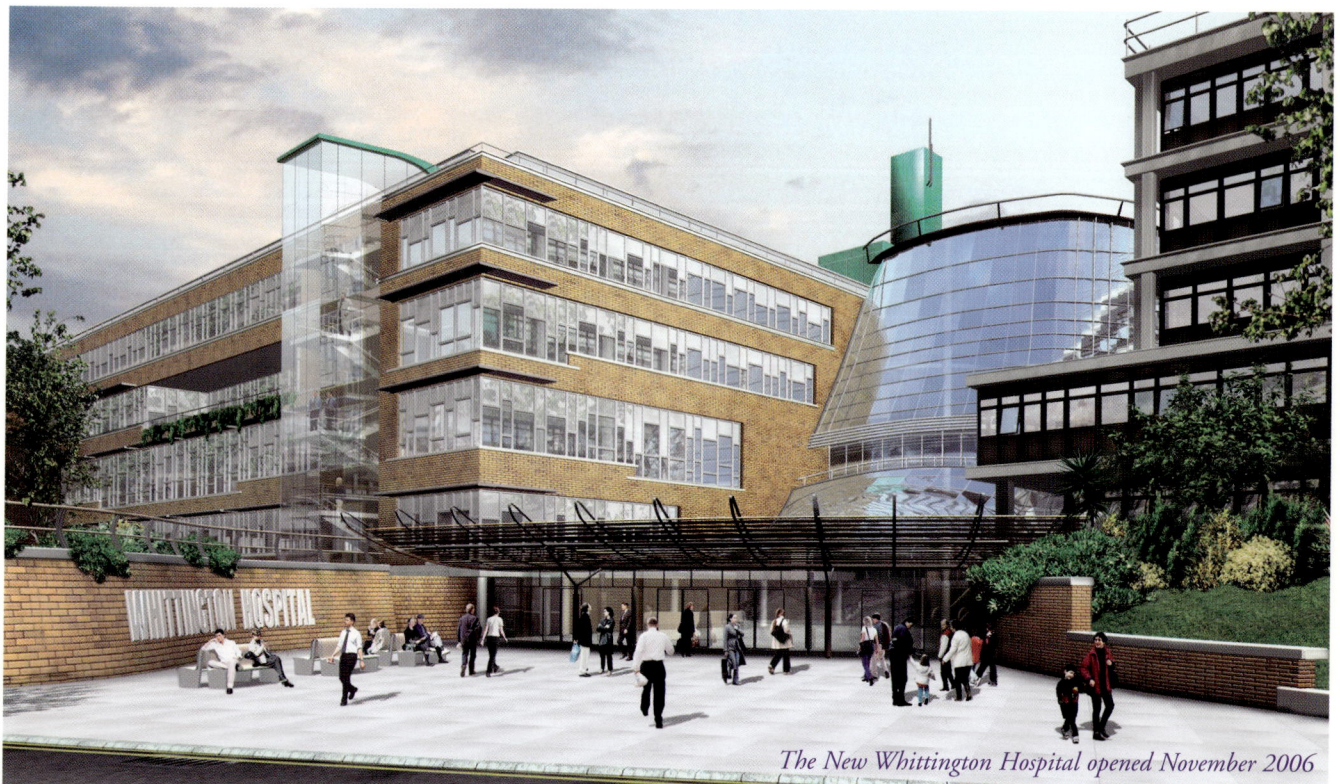

The New Whittington Hospital opened November 2006

Foreword

In these days of rapid and extensive changes in medicine and in our health services, great institutions, which may have served their community and their nations for generations, are disappearing at an alarming rate – and disappearing, moreover, without trace. As an example, my own hospital, the Westminster, is now a luxury block of apartments and there is nothing – not a blue plaque nor a little notice nor even a street name – to mark where the first of the great voluntary hospitals in this country, (founded in 1715), once proudly stood.

The Royal Northern was one such great hospital; loved and respected by the citizens of a large, densely populated and somewhat deprived area of North London, as well as being an important centre of undergraduate and postgraduate teaching. It attracted a consultant staff of international stature; men such as Lord Horder and Sir Lancelot Barrington-Ward. A duet of its surgeons, Hamilton Bailey and Robert McNeill Love, made publishing history with their textbooks and their most popular one is still in print, under a succession of eminent editors.

The closure of the Royal Northern in 1992 might well have meant the rapid loss of communal memory of this great institution. Fortunately, Dr Albert Rinsler, retired general practitioner, medical historian and himself a North Londoner, has rendered a great service by writing this interesting and beautifully illustrated history. He describes not only the changes in the sites and the fabric of the hospital, but also provides fascinating vignettes about its staff, both medical and non-medical, the famous and less famous among them. He also has preserved for us much archival material that would otherwise have been difficult to access.

I enjoyed reading this book in manuscript. I am sure everyone with an interest in medical history, and any North Londoner, will enjoy it too!

Professor Harold Ellis CBE DM MCh FRCS
Emeritus Professor of Surgery, University of London

Acknowledgements

The material for this book is partly derived from an exhibition, *A History of the Royal Northern Hospital*, which was originally displayed in the Great Northern Building of the Whittington Hospital. It is planned that the display will be relocated in the new wing of the Whittington Hospital.

I would like to thank GlaxoSmithKline, the Wellcome Library, London and the Whittington Hospital, (Colposcopy Fund and the History Fund) for their generous donations which made the production of this book possible.

I should also like to thank UCL Media Resources for their considerable expertise, patience and help with the graphic design of this book.

Last but not least, I would also like to acknowledge the excellent assistance in proof-reading by Deborah Goodhart, Head of Communications, Whittington Hospital and Pamela Kent, Friend of the Whittington Hospital.

Albert Rinsler

Albert Rinsler

Contents

Foundation of the Royal Northern Hospital – 1856

1

The Royal Northern Hospital owes its origin to one man, Sherard Freeman Statham. He was born on 17 May 1826 in Stone, near Aylesbury; his father was the Reverend Samuel Freeman Statham, then a curate. Sherard's mother was Jemima, the daughter of a wealthy London merchant, Joseph Travers. The marriage enriched her husband by some £30,000. They had three sons and four daughters, Sherard Statham was the second son and fourth child. His younger brother, John Lee Statham, became dental surgeon to the original Great Northern Hospital. A cousin, Hugh Worthington Statham (1809–1892) was Medical Attendant (Apothecary) to the Foundling Hospital and had the great honour of being elected Master of the Society of Apothecaries of London.

Sherard Statham entered University College London to study medicine. In 1846 he went on to win a Silver Medal for Medicine and in the following year he gained the University Gold Medal in the final MB, achieving a first in Medicine. In 1851 he passed the London FRCS and in the same year was appointed assistant surgeon to University College Hospital, London. However, an early promising career came to an abrupt end because of a scandal which involved some very foolish behaviour in the operating theatre. Statham had taken an active interest in the training of junior medical staff and medical students in the administration of chloroform. His manner, however, was regarded as brusque and even uncouth at times. On 21 May 1856, a special meeting of the Medical Committee at University College Hospital took place to consider a complaint against his conduct. This took the form of a letter to the Chairman

To Professor Ellis, Dean of the Faculty of Medicine

15 May 1856

I am deeply pained at being compelled to direct your attention to the conduct of a colleague… the behaviour of Mr Statham, the Junior Assistant Surgeon, in the Theatre of the hospital during the performance of some operations by me on Wednesday last, the 14th instant.

Whilst assisting Mr Footman the Assistant Medical Officer in administrating chloroform to a patient on whom I was about performing a dangerous capital operation, and who showed some reluctance to inhaling the Vapour, (chloroform) Mr Statham striking the patient in the side said to him "fill your bloody chest" and afterwards during the same or other operation used the same expression "bloody" in a similar sense.

On the same day, as I was about operating for fistula-in-ano, as the patient, a man, lay naked on the table, Mr Statham gave his bare buttocks a slap with the palm of his hand in an unseemly manner, exciting a laugh from the class.

Such language and such behaviour is in my opinion strongly to be deprecated when employed by an officer connected with an Educational Establishment as it sets a bad example to the Students. But it is especially objectionable, on so serious an occasion during the performance of important Surgical operations in public when in addition to the bad effects that the employment that the coarse expressions and vulgar behaviour must necessarily have upon the class, they must excite painful feeling in the minds of the strangers present, not infrequently consisting of friends of the patient and are, to say the least, disturbing to me who as the operator bears the whole responsibility of the case.

…I feel that I have now no alternative but to bring the matter before the proper authorities of the College and to request that you will adopt the necessary means to prevent a repetition of such conduct which is prejudicial to the dignity of the College and the interest of the School as it is disagreeable to myself.

I am etc (signed) John Erichsen

Letter from John Erichsen, Professor of Surgery, to the Chairman of the Medical Committee

of the Medical Committee from Mr John Erichsen, Professor of Surgery at University College Hospital. Statham did not deny his conduct and, at a meeting of University College Council, the case against Sherard Statham was considered, and a unanimous resolution was carried. The Hospital Committee and the Medical Committee approved the proposal of the Council to remove Statham from his post. On 28 May 1856, Statham was no longer Assistant Surgeon to University College Hospital.

Sherard Statham was thirty years old, but his dismissal did not deter him. He was interested in public health measures and aware of the needs of the poor of North London which were quite inadequate. Shortly after leaving University College Hospital in 1856, he founded, financed and organised a small independent hospital, which was called the Great Northern Hospital, situated at Kings Cross.

A house was leased at 11 York Road (now York Way), Kings Cross and on 30 June 1856 the Great Northern Hospital opened its doors. At that time no convenient hospital accommodation existed for the 270,000 inhabitants of the neighbourhood which bordered on King's Cross. The catchment area included Islington, Camden Town, Somers Town, Kentish Town, Highgate and Hampstead.

Sadly, Sherard Statham died of pulmonary tuberculosis on 12 June 1858 at the early age of 32, and is buried in the family tomb at Stone in Buckinghamshire.

The first Committee meeting included the following statement:

This Hospital is open to the Sick Poor to the extent of its means free of letters of recommendation or any other form of admission.

The management of the Hospital is in the hands of Committee, chosen annually from the general body of the Governors.

A donation of Ten Guineas, or an annual subscription of One Guinea, constitutes Governor.

For the convenience of the Labouring Poor, attendance of one or more of the Chief Medical Officers is given every day throughout the year, from Twelve to Two o'clock; while urgent cases are attended to at all hours.

Every effort is made to prevent delay in dispensing the Medicines prescribed.

A Maternity Charity is established in connection with the Institution for the attendance of poor married women at their own homes. Some or all of the Medical Officers will meet to consult in all urgent cases.

The first general report of the hospital commented:

The situation York Road, King's Cross has many recommendations. Placed at the junction of four extensive parishes, in a densely populated and poor neighbourhood, and in the immediate vicinity of the Great Northern Railway Station and the New Cattle Market, it is calculated to afford Hospital accommodation for thousands of our poorer fellow creatures who have been hitherto, in this respect, less favoured than the inhabitants of almost every other district in the Metropolis.

Great Northern Hospital, Caledonian Road, 1864–1888

2

In 1861 the Metropolitan Railway Company required the hospital premises at King's Cross, for an extension of their railway. This was to build an underground loop-line to the Great Northern line, King's Cross. An Act of Parliament of that year (1861) made it necessary for the hospital to find an alternative property. During this period, the hospital was in dire financial straits, so the enforced move was a blessing in disguise. After much bartering, a sum of £1,750 was agreed and the Railway Company made a house available for the hospital in Pentonville Road, for the temporary use of out-patients and accident cases. In 1862, the Spinal Hospital in Portland Road was amalgamated with the Great Northern Hospital and this site was temporarily used for in-patients. The money received from the Metropolitan Railway as compensation, enabled the hospital to discharge its debts and to purchase in 1863, a house in the Caledonian Road, at the corner of Twyford Street, Islington. At the end of 1867, the hospital had gained possession of three houses between Twyford Street and Stanmore Street, thereby increasing its facilities.

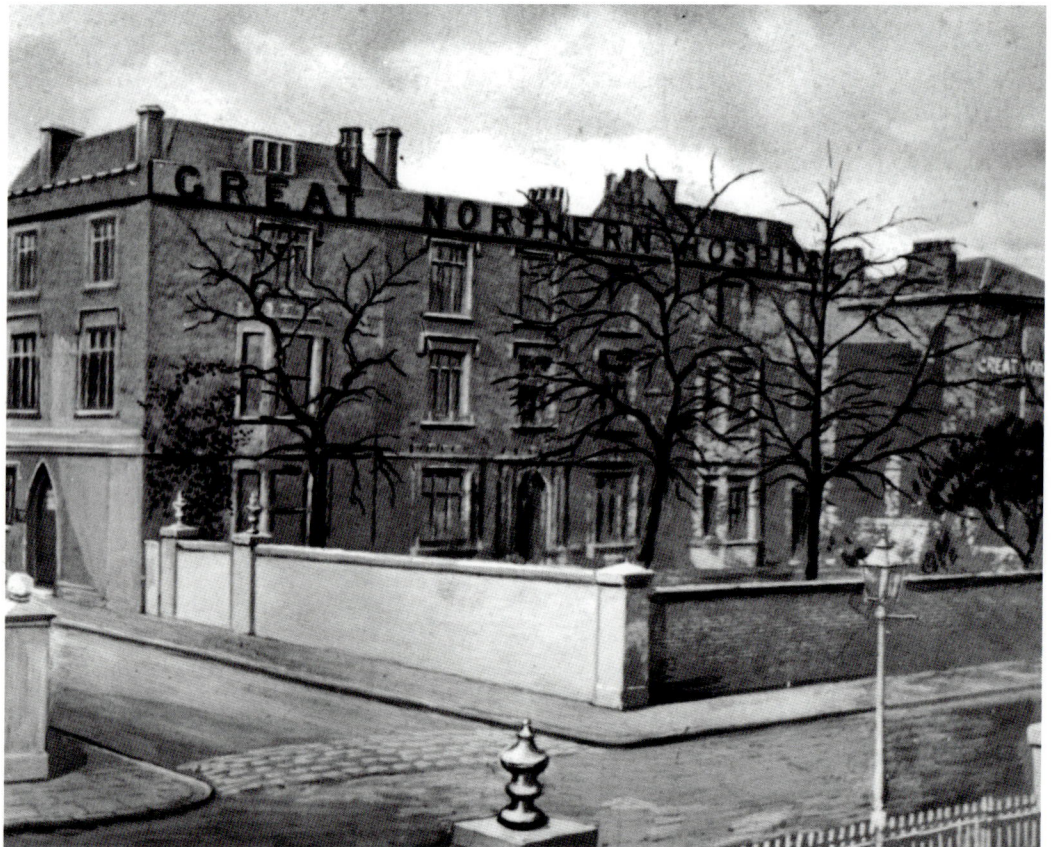

The Great Northern Hospital at Caledonian Road, 1864–1888.

Courtesy Islington Local History Collection

The Lancet Investigation

INTO THE

ADMINISTRATION OF THE OUT-PATIENT DEPARTMENT OF THE LONDON HOSPITALS

GREAT NORTHERN HOSPITAL, CALEDONIAN ROAD

This hospital is situated at a considerable distance from any other, and is in the centre of a large and populous district, many of the inhabitants belonging to the artisan and labouring classes. The number of out-patients attended last year was as follows:–

	New.	Old.	Total.
Physicians' cases	7989 ...	14973 ...	22962
Surgeons' cases	3987 ...	10223 ...	14210
Dental	5129 ...	...	5129
Diseases of the eye	473 ...	870 ...	1343
Diseases of women and children ...	362 ...	499 ...	861
Casualties	5324 ...	10876 ...	16200
	23264 ...	37441 ...	60705

The patients are received in a building which was formerly the hospital. As negotiations are pending the renewal of the lease, the rooms have not been specially prepared for the reception of the patients. There is, however, ample accommodation, in six separate waiting-rooms, for about 200 patients. The average number present at any one time is about 125. The patients are admitted from nine to ten A.M. Casualties are received by the house surgeon throughout the day, and the physicians extend the time to patients from the country. The porter frequently refuses admission to persons finely dressed, and those who appear able to contribute something are requested to pay 2s. 6d. to the charity, by doing which they secure the privilege of being examined first. The average receipts from this source are about £1 per week. It is also to be noted that the whole of the inhabitants are thoroughly canvassed for subscriptions, and that a very considerable amount is obtained from the working classes, in sums of 5s. and under. After the admission of the special cases, the males and females are seen, the porter selecting the feeble and more obviously serious cases for early entrance. The patients are ordered to remain in the waiting-rooms; but the ladies are somewhat hard to keep in order, and a threat is posted up that if not obedient the surgeon 'will not see one of them'. Every patient is examined privately. One only is permitted to remain within a reasonable distance of the consulting-room door, in order to be ready when summoned by a bell. This is as it should be.

The dispensing is for the present carried on in a kitchen, very roughly fitted up, but provided with sufficient drugs. About three quarts of cod-liver oil, one ounce of quinine, and two ounces of cinchonine are used per day. The bottles are received and given out through a trap-door, which cannot be kept open.

On the whole we have great satisfaction in speaking of the out-patient department of this hospital. It presents a model which older institutions might usefully imitate. It is doing good work well; and we hope that the funds will be forthcoming to fit up the building and dispensary in a proper way.

Extract from The Lancet *13 November 1869*

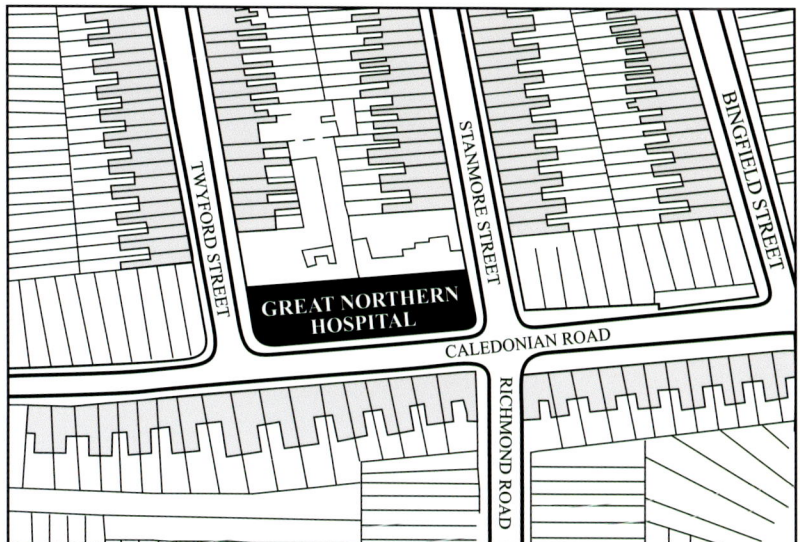

Map of the area, based on an Ordnance Survey Map of 1871

The Doctor, by Luke Fildes RA (1843–1927) and Dr Gustavus Murray MD (1831–1887)

3

The Doctor is a great masterpiece of late Victorian painting by Luke Fildes RA and is probably his greatest work. There is circumstantial evidence that the inspiration for the painting was derived from an incident in the artist's life. One Victorian doctor is closely connected with the painting; Dr Gustavus Murray, a consultant obstetrician at the Great Northern Hospital who probably played a crucial role in its creation.

In 1890 Henry Tate commissioned the artist Luke Fildes, but gave him a free hand in the choice of his subject. The painting was finished in 1891 and was purchased by Tate for his new National Gallery of British Art at Millbank (later known as the Tate Gallery). *The Doctor* was exhibited at the Royal Academy in 1891 and has hung in the Tate Gallery since 1897. The painting is a large oil on canvas some 7½ft x 5½ft and shows an interior based on a humble fisherman's cottage A full size reproduction of the cottage was built in a corner of the studio in Fildes' house, in Melbury Road, Kensington. Geoffrey, one of

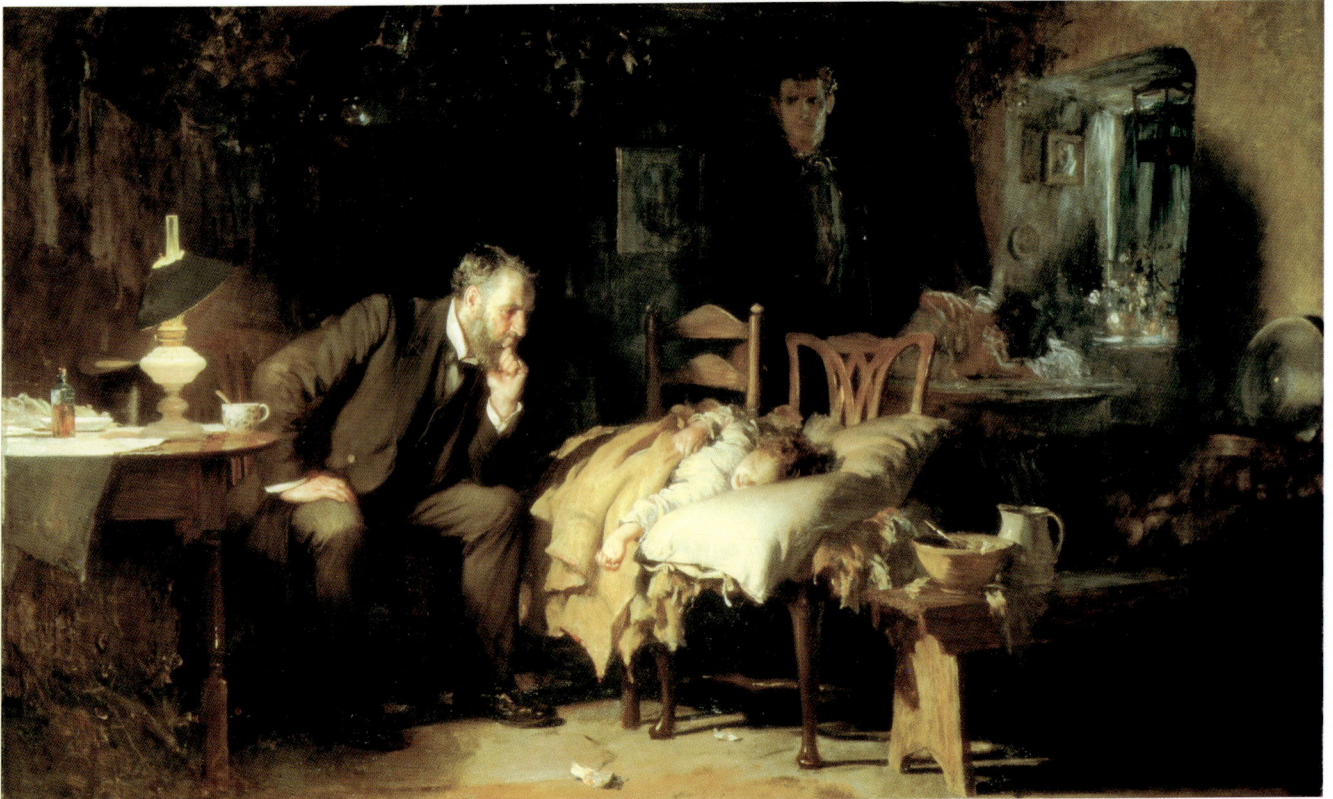

The Doctor 1891 by Luke Fildes RA. 166.3cm x 231.9cm. ©Tate, London 2005

Fildes' children is thought to be the model for the sick child. The doctor portrayed in the painting is looking thoughtfully at the sick child who appears to be pale and ill. The father is in shadow looking grave: the mother is seated at the table, with her head buried in her arms and her hands clasped.

The painting was very popular in its day. An engraving published by Agnew's of London produced a large sale in the United Kingdom and over one million copies were sold in the United States. In 1947, to commemorate the centenary of the American Medical Association, the United States Postal Service reproduced *The Doctor* as a three cent stamp. In 1970, Dominica produced it as an eight cent stamp on the centenary of the British Red Cross.

Henry Tate (1819–1899)

The son of a Lancashire clergyman, Henry Tate came to Liverpool at the age of thirteen as an apprentice to a grocer. By the age of twenty he had branched out on his own and had become the owner of six successful grocery shops.

The new firm of Henry Tate & Sons undertook the construction of a sugar refinery in Liverpool which was opened in 1872, and some six years later the Thames refinery was built in Silvertown, London, mainly for the manufacture of cube sugar. Tate & Lyle was created in 1921 by the amalgamation of Henry Tate & Sons and Abram Lyle (Lyles Golden Syrup).

Tate was munificent to British art and was a most generous philanthropist to education, and medical care in Liverpool. He died in 1899 at the age of eighty.

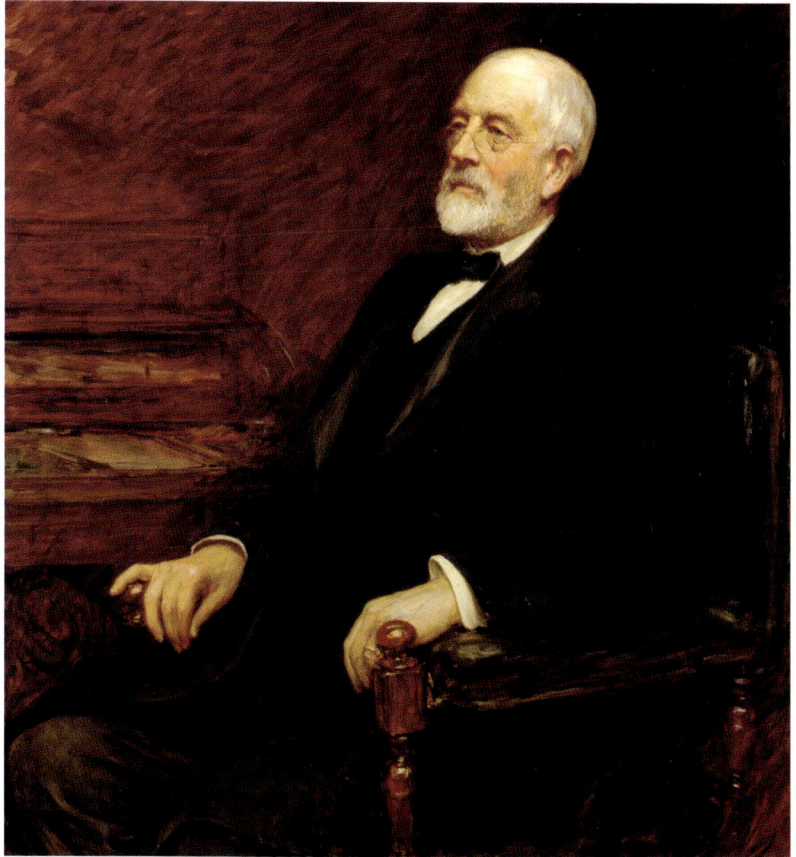

Henry Tate 1897, by Sir Hubert von Herkomer RA (1849–1914).

©Tate, London 2005

Luke Fildes RA (1843–1927)

Samuel Luke Fildes was born in 1843 in a poor district of Liverpool where his father James Fildes kept a large lodging house for seamen. Fildes' grandmother, Mrs Mary Fildes, was a very remarkable woman and had taken part in the Reform Movement. On 16 August 1819 an estimated crowd of 60,000 people, men, women and children had assembled at St Peter's Field, Manchester. The meeting was a protest at a time of economic depression. Mary Fildes was on the platform with 'Orator' Hunt, MP for Preston. The authorities panicked and ordered the cavalrymen to charge the crowd (Peterloo

Massacre), and in the mêlée Mary Fildes was seriously wounded by a sabre slash. She eventually left Manchester for a more sheltered life in Chester. When young Fildes was eleven years old, his grandmother took him to live with her but the reason for this is obscure. There, he started to develop his interest in art. He joined the Warrington School of Art, where he met his future brother-in-law and lifelong friend Henry Woods.

In 1863 aged twenty, Fildes was awarded a scholarship at a school for industrial design in South Kensington. His ambition was to become a book illustrator and by good fortune his work came to the notice of Millais who introduced him to Charles Dickens; Fildes drew the illustrations for *Edwin Drood*. By now Fildes was regarded as one of the most able book illustrators in the country.

In the early 1870s Fildes returned to oil painting. One that brought him fame was *Applicants for Admission to a Casual Ward*, which hangs in the Royal Holloway College. In 1874 he married Fanny, the pretty sister of his best friend and fellow student Henry Woods. She later became an ARA, her brother an RA. Luke Fildes was elected RA in 1887 and was knighted in 1906; he died in 1927 at the age of eighty-four.

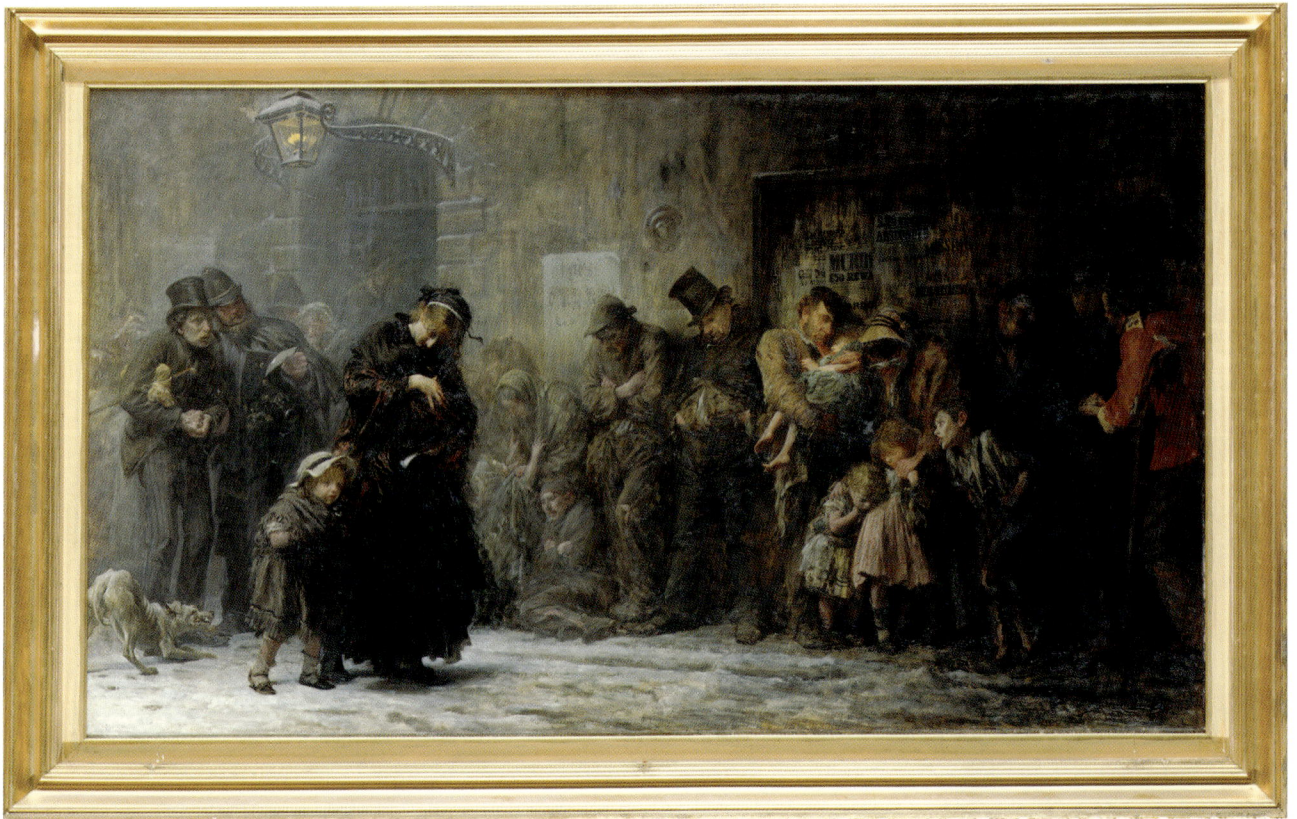

Applicants for Admission to a Casual Ward 1874, by Luke Fildes RA 137.1cm x 243.7cm.
Picture supplied courtesy of the Royal Holloway University of London

The Fildes had seven children, two girls and five boys. Two sons achieved distinction – one in commerce and the other in medicine. Luke Val Fildes, 1879–1971, had a long and notable career with Unilever and was his father's biographer. Sir Paul Fildes FRS (1882–1971) was a distinguished medical scientist and is regarded as one of the foremost microbiologists of the twentieth century.

1877 was an eventful year for Luke Fildes who had become well known and very successful. The family had moved into their newly built very large house in Melbury Road, Kensington. Philip, their first-born, had become very ill just before Christmas 1877 and died on Christmas morning. It is very probable that this event had a considerable influence on the creation of *The Doctor*. Luke Val Fildes writes in his father's biography:

'The character and bearing of their doctor throughout the time of their anxiety, made a deep impression on my parents. Dr Murray became a symbol of professional devotion which would one day inspire The Doctor…

…The Doctor *had been on my father's mind ever since Dr Murray watched over Philip.'*

The death certificate, signed by Dr Murray, states the cause of death as convulsions, which was a very commonly reported cause of death. Meningitis would come high in

the differential diagnosis in the child's illness and death. From data derived from the Registrar-General's report of 1877, the mortality rate for children under five years of age in London in 1877 was 25 per cent and under one, 14.6 per cent.

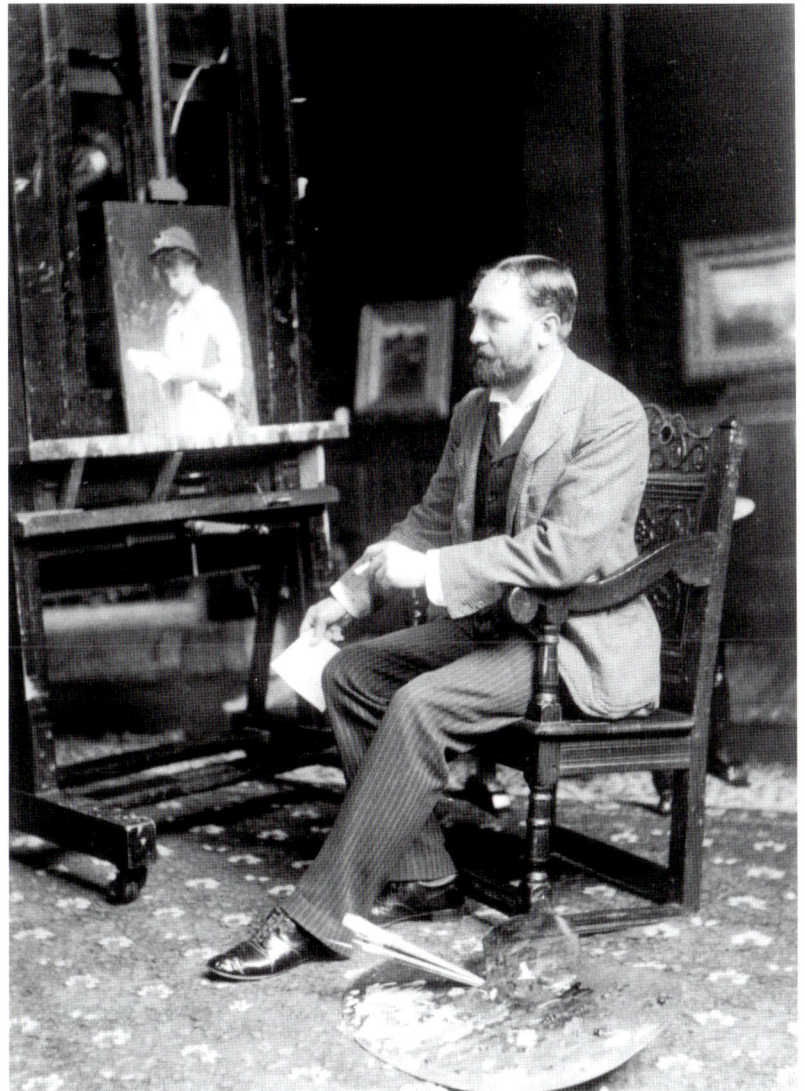

Luke Fildes RA 1887, photograph by Ralph Winwood Robinson.
Courtesy Royal Photographic Society Collection,
National Museum for Photography, Film & TV, Bradford Collection

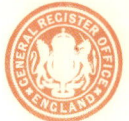

CERTIFIED COPY OF AN ENTRY OF DEATH

Given at the GENERAL REGISTER OFFICE, SOMERSET HOUSE, LONDON.

The fee for this certificate is 8s. 0d.
When application is made by post a
handling fee is payable in addition.

Application Number......PAS 83512/61

REGISTRATION DISTRICT _Kensington_

___1877.___ **DEATH** in the Sub-district of _Kensington Town_ in the _County of Middlesex_

No.	When and where died	Name and surname	Sex	Age	Occupation	Cause of death	Signature, description, and residence of informant	When registered	Signature of registrar
	Columns :— 1	2	3	4	5	6	7	8	9
390	Twenty fifth December 1877 1 Melbury Road	Philip Luke Fildes	Male	1 year	Son of Samuel Luke Fildes known as Luke Fildes Artist Painter	Dentition 1 month Convulsions 5 days Exhaustion Certified by G. Murray M.D	Luke Fildes Father Present at the death 1 Melbury Road	Twenty-seventh December 1877	C.R. Barnes Registrar

CERTIFIED to be a true copy of an entry in the certified copy of a Register of Deaths in the District above mentioned.
Given at the GENERAL REGISTER OFFICE, SOMERSET HOUSE, LONDON, under the Seal of the said Office, the _31st_ day of _July_ 19 _69_

DA 549486

This certificate is issued in pursuance of the Births and Deaths Registration Act 1953.
Section 34 provides that any certified copy of an entry purporting to be sealed or stamped with the seal of the General Register Office shall be received as evidence of the birth or death to which it relates without any further or other proof of the entry, and no certified copy purporting to be given in the said Office shall be of any force or effect unless it is sealed or stamped as aforesaid.
CAUTION.—Any person who (1) falsifies any of the particulars on this certificate, or (2) uses a falsified certificate as true, knowing it to be false, is liable to prosecution.

Death certificate of Philip Fildes, signed by Dr Murray.

Office of National Statistics. Crown copyright material, reproduced with the permission of the Controller

Dr Gustavus Charles Philip Murray MD (1831–1887)

Dr Gustavus Murray was born in Trinidad, the youngest son of the Honourable Edward Murray, Marshal of the Courts of Trinidad and Registrar of Slaves. Because of his poor health, Dr Murray's general education was in private schools in England. He decided to study medicine and enrolled as a student at King's College Hospital, London, then in Portugal Street. He qualified MRCS LRCP in 1856 and early in his career became interested in obstetrics. After qualifying he went as a postgraduate at the Vienna General Lying-in Hospital, where the famous Dr Ignaz Semmelweiss (1818–1865) had done his great pioneering work on puerperal fever.

In 1856 Dr Murray married Fanny Yearsley of Cheltenham. Her uncle, James Yearsley 1805–1869 was a pioneer of oto-laryngology. He founded the Metropolitan Ear and Throat Hospital, Fitzroy Square, London and was also one of the founders of the Medical Directory.

Dr Murray was very closely associated with the Obstetrical Society of London, founded in 1858. He successively became Secretary and Treasurer. In 1907 the Society was absorbed with other medical societies to become the Royal Society of Medicine.

In 1860, Dr Murray journeyed up to Edinburgh and obtained his MD and in 1863 he applied for the post of Physician Accoucheur (consultant obstetrician) at the Great Northern Hospital, Caledonian Road. The Medical Committee unanimously recommended him for the post which he held until his relatively early death in 1887 at the age of fifty-six.

Dr Murray was devoted to obstetrics and excelled in this specialty, which is reflected in an extract from his obituary in The Lancet:

'His manual dexterity was remarkable. His judgement in the conduct of cases was excellent; never hurried or impatient, he would wait on natural effort, if that seemed best for any length of time; and if help was needed, he seemed always to give it at the right time and in the best way. These gifts and qualities made him highly successful and his advice and help was sought and greatly valued by large numbers of practitioners…'

The fulminating and fatal illness of their first-born son Philip must have been a harrowing ordeal for the Fildes, but they would have had the unstinting support of their very caring doctor. Although the doctor in the painting does not represent any one individual, the characterisation of care and devotion that he displays may well have been due to the memory of Dr Gustavus Murray.

In 1892, Mr Mitchell Banks MD FRCS, surgeon to the Liverpool Royal Infirmary, in an address to future medical students at Yorkshire College, Leeds said:

'…A library of books written in our honour would not do what this picture has done and will do for the medical profession in making the hearts of our fellow-men warm to us with confidence and affection…so that you may bring to bear upon your patients' cases not merely a knowledge of morbid anatomy and drugs, but also a knowledge of the ways of the world and of the inner working of men's lives …remember always to hold before you the ideal figure of Luke Fildes' picture, and be at once gentle men and gentle doctors.'

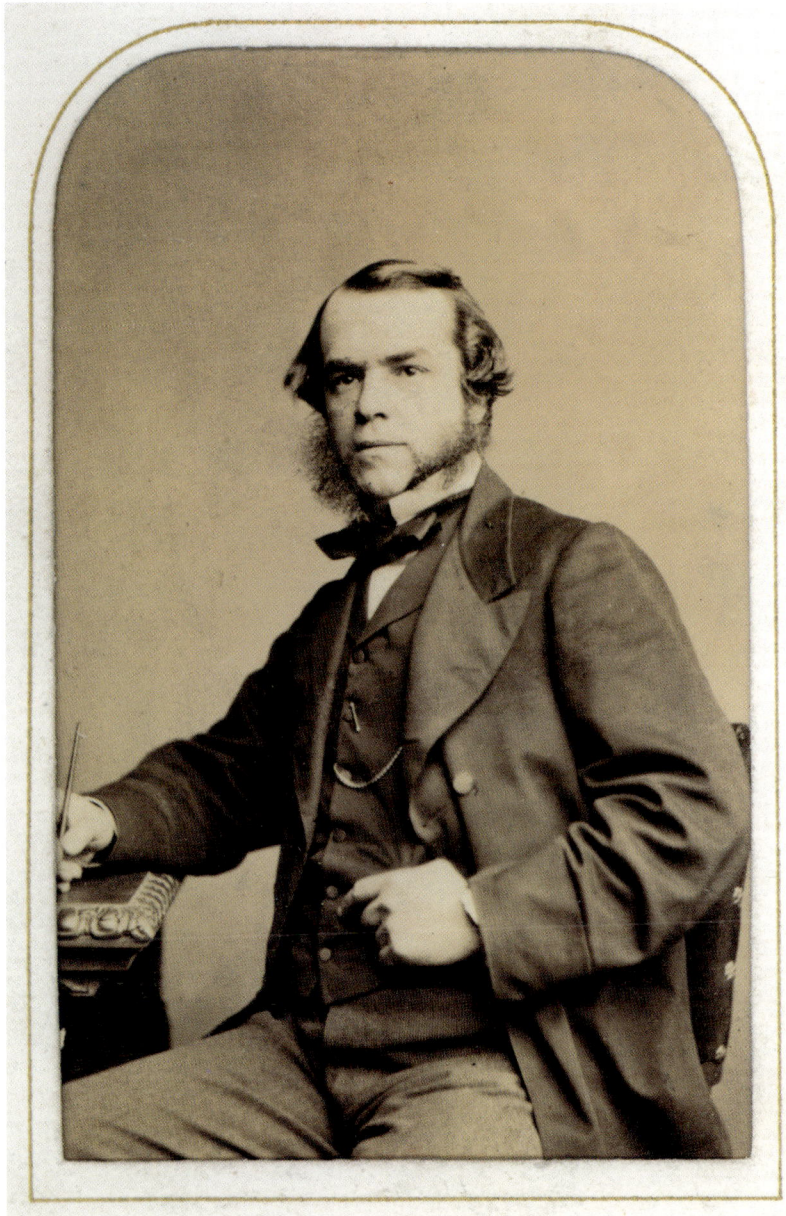

Photograph of Dr Gustavus Murray MD, 1867.
By kind permission of the Royal Society of Medicine

Robert Bridges OM DLit LLD FRCP (1844–1930)

4

Robert Seymour Bridges was born at Walmer, Kent on 23 October 1844 and was descended from a long line of Kentish farmers. From Eton, where 'he studied, read and wrote verses constantly', he went to Corpus Christi College, Oxford and took an arts degree. Leaving Oxford, he travelled abroad in Europe and the Middle East.

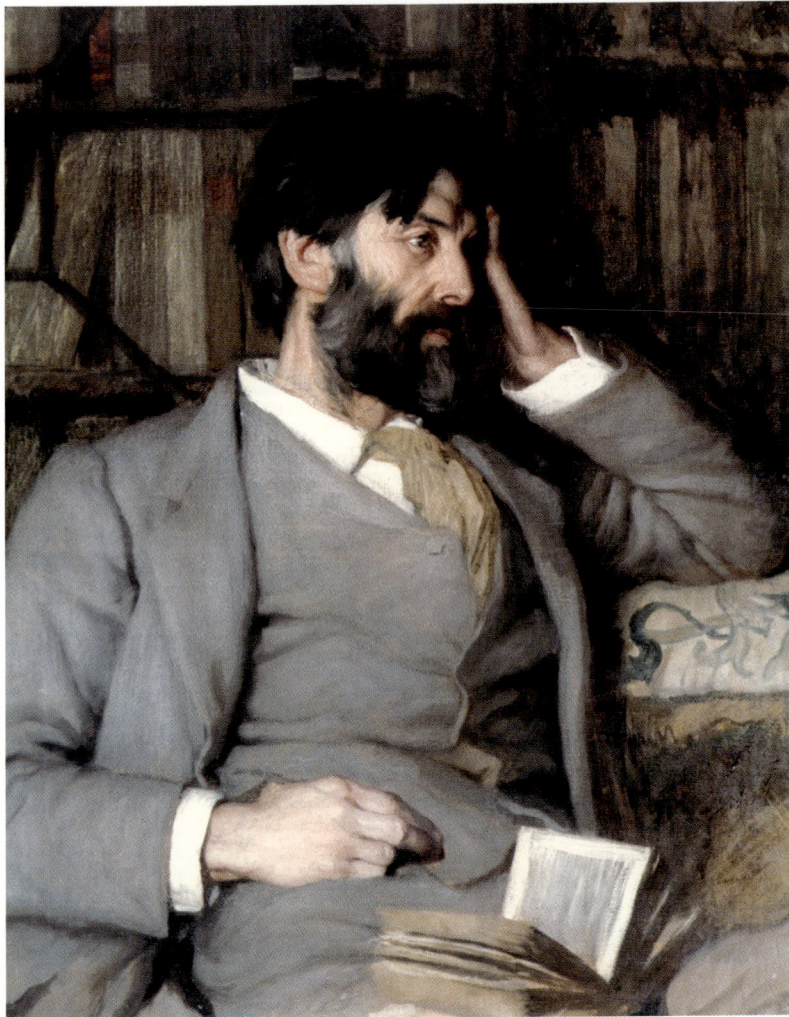

In 1869 at the age of twenty-five he decided to study medicine, and became a student at St. Bartholomew's Hospital. He graduated in 1874 MB (Oxon), aged thirty. During the year 1877–1878 he was one of three casualty physicians at Bartholomew's Hospital, and from his experiences he wrote *An Account of the Casualty Department*. It exposed an 'intolerable system' and Bridges estimated that he saw over 30,000 patients during his year with an average time of 1.28 minutes per patient! To this it was countered that the function of a Casualty Physician was not to attend and prescribe, but to act as a 'filter'. This very critical report of Robert Bridges ensured that he would never have another appointment at Bart's! A very distinguished physician Sir Walter Langdon Brown, warned a student audience 'the powers that be, do not appreciate irony, and youthful reformers still find it advisable to curb their tongues and pens'.

Dr Robert Bridges, portrait in oils, exhibited at the Royal Academy 1894. Charles Furse ARA 1868–1904.

Reproduced by kind permission of the Provost and Fellows of Eton College

In 1878 he was appointed physician to the out-patient department of the Great Northern Central Hospital, Caledonian Road, and in the same year he was appointed assistant physician to the Hospital for Sick Children, Great Ormond Street. In 1879 he was elected full physician to the in-patient department of the Great Northern Central Hospital.

In 1881, Dr Bridges unfortunately contracted pneumonia complicated by an empyema (a collection of pus in the pleural cavity). After convalescing in Italy, he resigned his post and retired from medicine at the early age of thirty-seven. It was always his intention to leave the profession and pursue his chosen career as a poet; fortunately he had ample means to do this. In 1900 the Royal College of Physicians honoured themselves by electing him a Fellow!

In 1913 his position in the world of letters was recognised by his appointment as Poet Laureate. His last but perhaps his greatest work was *The Testament of Beauty*, which was published on his eighty-fifth birthday.

His most distinguished honour was the Order of Merit, which he received in 1929. Robert Bridges died at his home in Boars Hill, Oxford in 1930, at the age of eighty-six.

Nightingales

Beautiful must be the mountains whence ye came.
And bright in the fruitful valleys the streams, wherefrom
Ye learn your song:
Where are the starry woods? O might I wander there
Among the flowers, which in the heavenly air
Bloom the year long!

Nay, barren are those mountains and spent the streams:
Our song is the voice of desire, that haunts our dreams,
A throe of the heart,
Whose pining visions, forbidden hopes profound,
No dying cadence nor long sigh can sound
For all our art.

Alone, aloud in the raptured ear of men
We pour our dark nocturnal secret; and then
As night is withdrawn
From these sweet-springing meads and bursting boughs of may,
Dream, while the innumerable choir of day
Welcome the dawn.

The Poetical Works of Robert Bridges with The Testament of Beauty Book V. *1936.*

By permission of Oxford University Press

William Adams FRCS (1820–1900)

5

William Adams was the son of James Adams, surgeon and governor of St Thomas' Hospital. In 1838 William Adams entered St Thomas' Hospital as a medical student. There he came under the influence of the very distinguished surgeon Joseph Henry Green FRCS FRS (1791–1863), who became his teacher and mentor. Among the latter's many appointments and attainments, he was elected President of The Royal College of Surgeons, became the first Professor of Surgery at King's College London, and was Professor of Anatomy at the Royal College of Art.

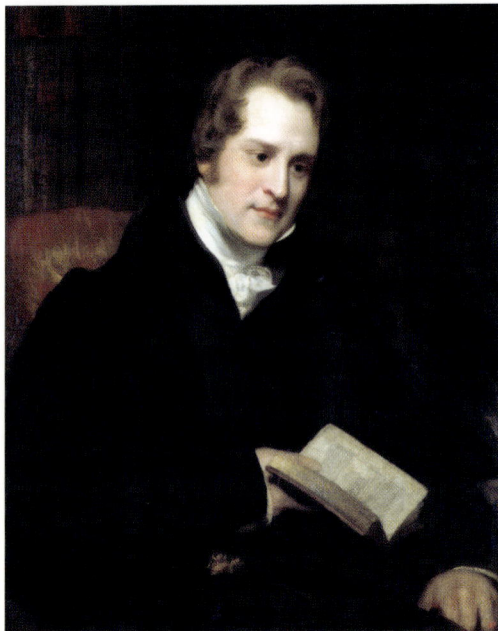

Joseph Henry Green. Oil on canvas by Thomas Phillips RA (1770–1845). Undated and unsigned.
Reproduced by kind permission of the President and Council of the Royal College of Surgeons of England

Adams qualified MRCS in 1842 and in the same year was appointed Curator of the Museum, at St Thomas' Hospital. He obtained the FRCS in 1851 and in 1854 joined Lane's Medical School, a private medical school near St George's Hospital. He lectured on Surgery and Hospital Practice, having Sir Thomas Spencer Wells MD FRCS (1818–1897) as a colleague. Spencer Wells was a renowned gynaecologist and designer of surgical instruments, including an artery forceps which bears his name.

Around 1854, Adams began to devote his attention, more particularly towards orthopaedic surgery and was appointed to the staff at the Royal Orthopaedic Hospital, Bloomsbury Square (later the Royal National Orthopaedic Hospital, Great Portland Street). He was also a consultant at the National Hospital for the Paralysed and Epileptic, Queen's Square. In 1858 Adams joined the staff of the Great Northern Hospital, King's Cross.

William Adams was the best known orthopaedic surgeon of his time in England. He had a particular interest in pathology and in the treatment of skeletal deformities. By 1869 the Great Northern Hospital had moved from Kings Cross to Caledonian Road and was known as the Great Northern Central Hospital. Here, Adams introduced the operation of subcutaneous osteotomy of the neck of the femur within the capsule of the hip joint. He designed a long

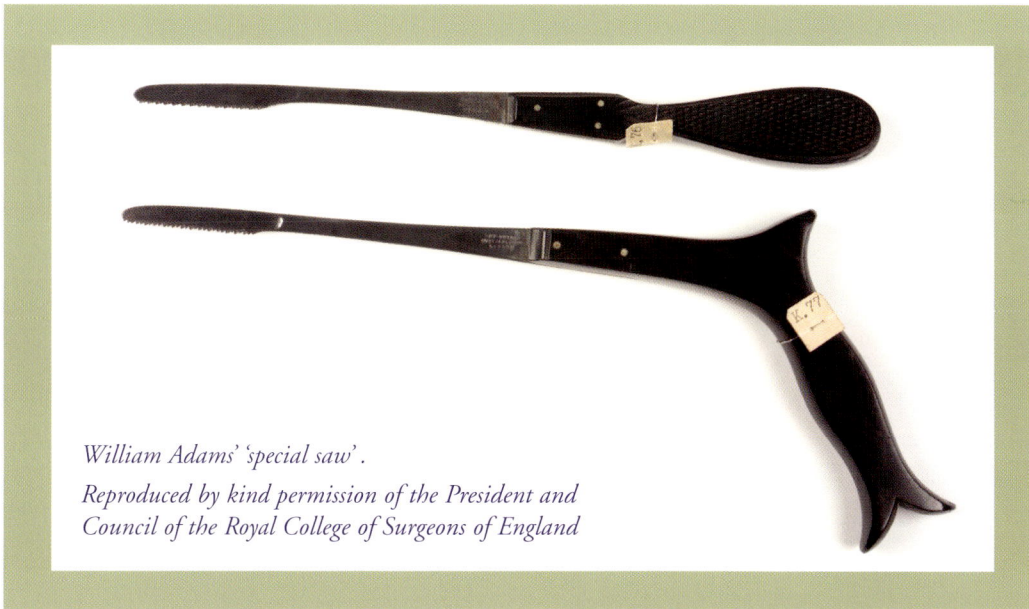

William Adams' 'special saw'.
Reproduced by kind permission of the President and
Council of the Royal College of Surgeons of England

handled tenotomy knife with a short blade, for division of the muscles and the opening of the joint capsule; this was through a very small stab wound prior to the osteotomy. Adams invented a special saw for dividing the femoral neck of the femur. This saw had a short cutting surface, 3/8inch wide with a long shank and handle; 'my little thaw' as he always called it (*he had a well marked lisp*).

Adams brought into prominence the treatment of Dupuytren's contracture by subcutaneous division of fibrous bands in the palm. (Baron Guillaume Dupuytren 1777–1835, a famous French surgeon).

Adams published a treatise on spinal curvature, advocating the use of postural and instrumental correction of scoliosis. He was awarded the Jacksonian Prize of the Royal College of Surgeons in 1864 for an essay on '*Club Foot, its causes, pathology and treatment*'.

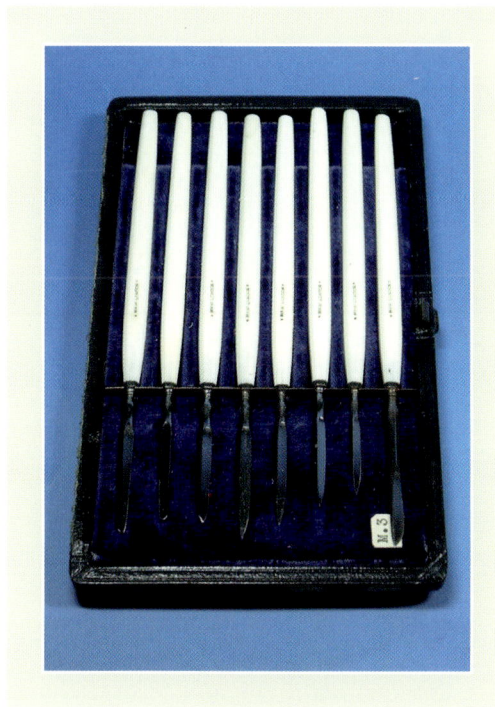

William Adams' variety of tenotomy knives.
Reproduced by kind permission of the President and
Council of the Royal College of Surgeons of England

A case of breach of promise
Adams v Russell (Extract)
In the Court of Exchequer.*

*Court of Exchequer was a court in Great Britain dealing with matters of Revenue, now merged with the King's or Queen's Bench.

In 1863, Adams successfully defended a suit for breach of promise brought by a Miss Russell, a patient of William Adams. It seems that her mother, Mrs Emily Russell was the instigator of the case and a main witness for the plaintiff. It also appears that Mrs Russell was impecunious and was in considerable debt. Much of the evidence by Mrs Russell was that Adams by implication was going to marry Miss Russell. Mrs Russell also stated that on one occasion Adams had put his arms round Miss Russell's waist. Mr Adams in his evidence had told Miss Russell that he was married. Miss Russell according to her mother did not believe him, and thought that he was teasing. In fact, Mr Adams married in August 1847 and at the time of the trial, had a wife and three children. Mrs Russell's insinuations against William Adams could not be supported. The judge, Lord Chief Justice Pollock, in his summing up, appeared to have believed Adams with other corroborating testimony, that Adams had told the girl that he was married nor did he think that Adams had seduced the girl. The jury was out for two hours but could not agree, and with some impatience from the judge they were sent back to deliberate. They then returned after fifteen minutes.

The foreman: "This is our verdict as the plaintiff has not made out her case to our entire satisfaction we are necessitated to find a verdict for the defendant. Verdict for defendant accordingly".

Extract from notes of Court report.

By kind permission of the Royal Society of Medicine

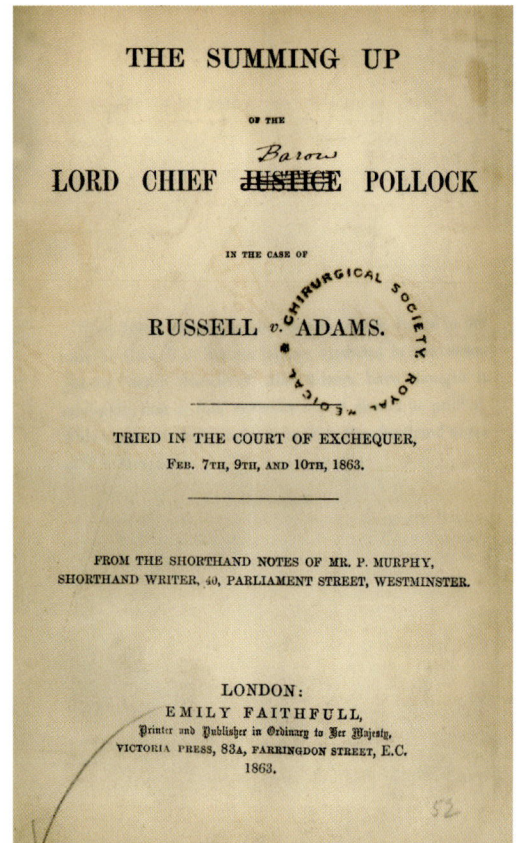

THE SUMMING UP

OF THE

LORD CHIEF ~~JUSTICE~~ *Baron* POLLOCK

IN THE CASE OF

RUSSELL *v.* ADAMS.

ROYAL MEDICAL & CHIRURGICAL SOCIETY

TRIED IN THE COURT OF EXCHEQUER,
FEB. 7TH, 9TH, AND 10TH, 1863.

FROM THE SHORTHAND NOTES OF MR. P. MURPHY,
SHORTHAND WRITER, 40, PARLIAMENT STREET, WESTMINSTER.

LONDON:
EMILY FAITHFULL,
Printer and Publisher in Ordinary to Her Majesty,
VICTORIA PRESS, 83A, FARRINGDON STREET, E.C.
1863.

Frontispiece of court report notes.
By kind permission of the Royal Society of Medicine

In 1890, William Adams retired from the Great Northern Central Hospital which had now moved to Holloway Road. He had lived and practised from his home at 5 Henrietta Street, Cavendish Square until 1896, when he moved to Loudon Road, St John's Wood.

His house in Henrietta Street eventually became the 'home' of the Royal College of Nursing. Adams died on 3 February 1900 aged eighty.

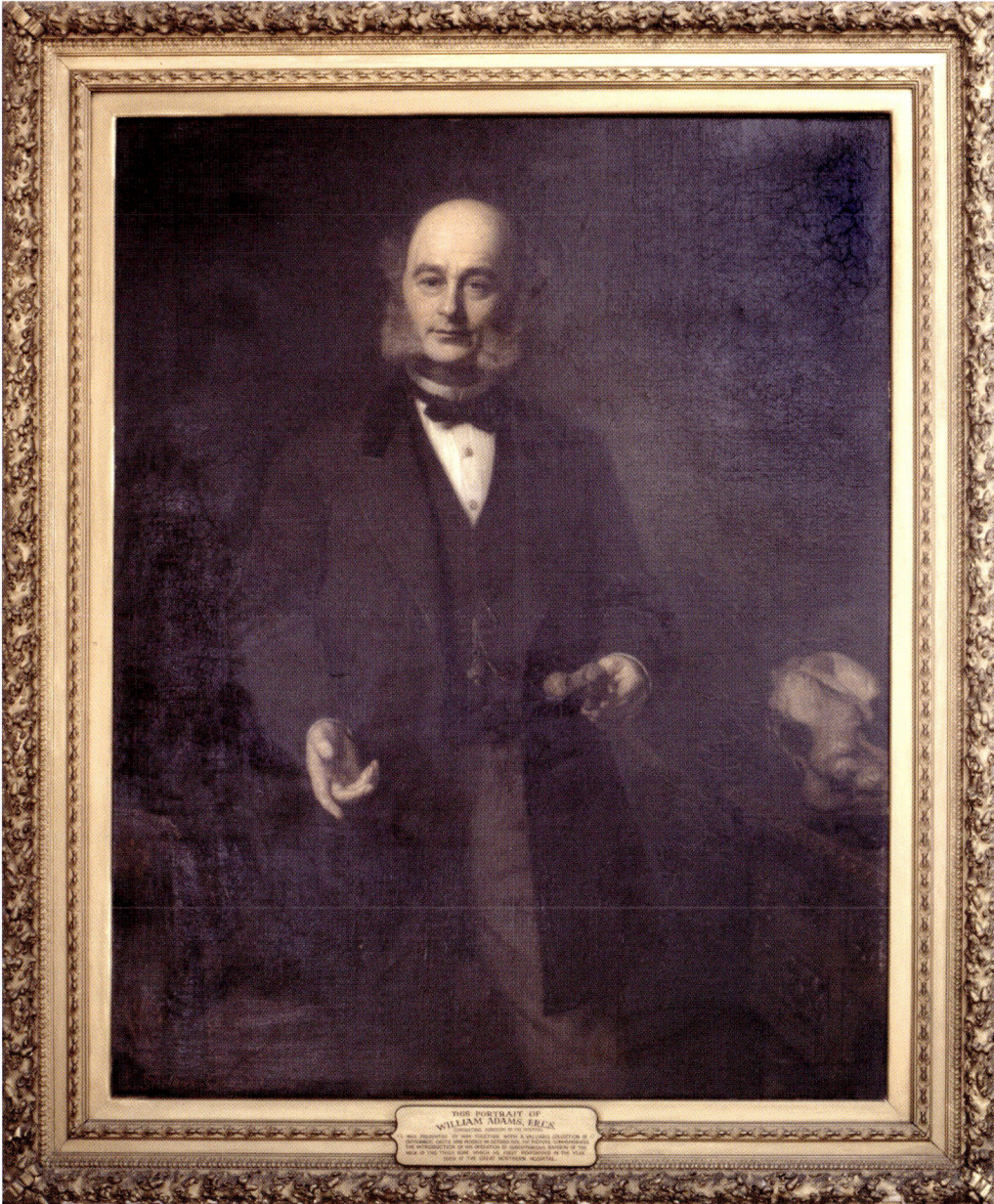

THIS PORTRAIT OF
WILLIAM ADAMS. F.R.C.S.
CONSULTING SURGEON TO THE HOSPITAL

WAS PRESENTED BY HIM TOGETHER WITH A VALUABLE COLLECTION OF
ORTHOPAEDIC CASTS AND MODELS IN OCTOBER 1895. THE PICTURE COMMEMORATES
THE INTRODUCTION OF HIS OPERATION OF SUBCUTANEOUS DIVISION OF THE
NECK OR THE THIGH BONE WHICH HE FIRST PERFORMED IN THE YEAR
1869 AT THE GREAT NORTHERN HOSPITAL

William Adams FRCS 1896, portrait in oils by Ernest Gustavo Gerardo RBA, (whereabouts of painting unknown).

Courtesy the Royal Northern Hospital Archives, Whittington Hospital

The Move to Holloway Road

6

The population was growing, but there was a lack of general hospital accommodation in North London. The consequence of this situation in 1883 was a proposal to establish another hospital, the Central Hospital for North London. However a joint meeting of both hospital committees decided that the best solution was to amalgamate. In 1884, the Great Northern Hospital became known as the Great Northern Central Hospital, which was still on the same site, in Caledonian Road. The total bed capacity was still only thirty-three beds but it was not possible

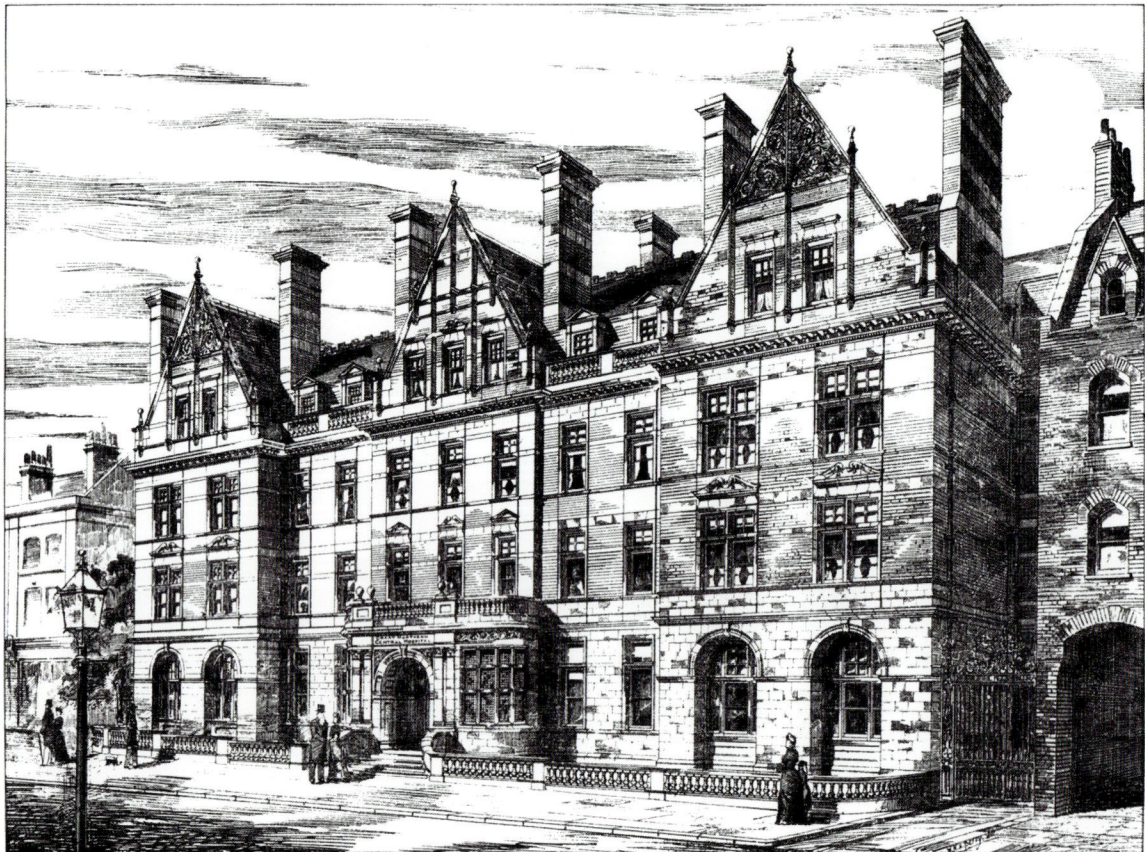

THE BUILDER, DECEMBER 25 1886

GREAT NORTHERN CENTRAL HOSPITAL.—Mr. Keith D. Young, F.R.I.B.A., and Mr. Henry Hall, A.R.I.B.A., Architects.

Architects sketch of proposed new building. The Builder *25 Dec 1886. Courtesy the London Metropolitan Archives, The Corporation of London*

to rebuild the hospital; there was now an urgent need to find a larger site. In December 1884 the purchase of a site in Holloway Road (Grove House estate) was obtained for £7,250. The architects for the winning plans were Messrs Young and Hall. The estimated total costs for building were £45,000, but after the purchase of the site the Committee was left with only £2,300 in the Building Fund for development! A public appeal was organised; local musical and dramatic societies organised performances to raise funds.

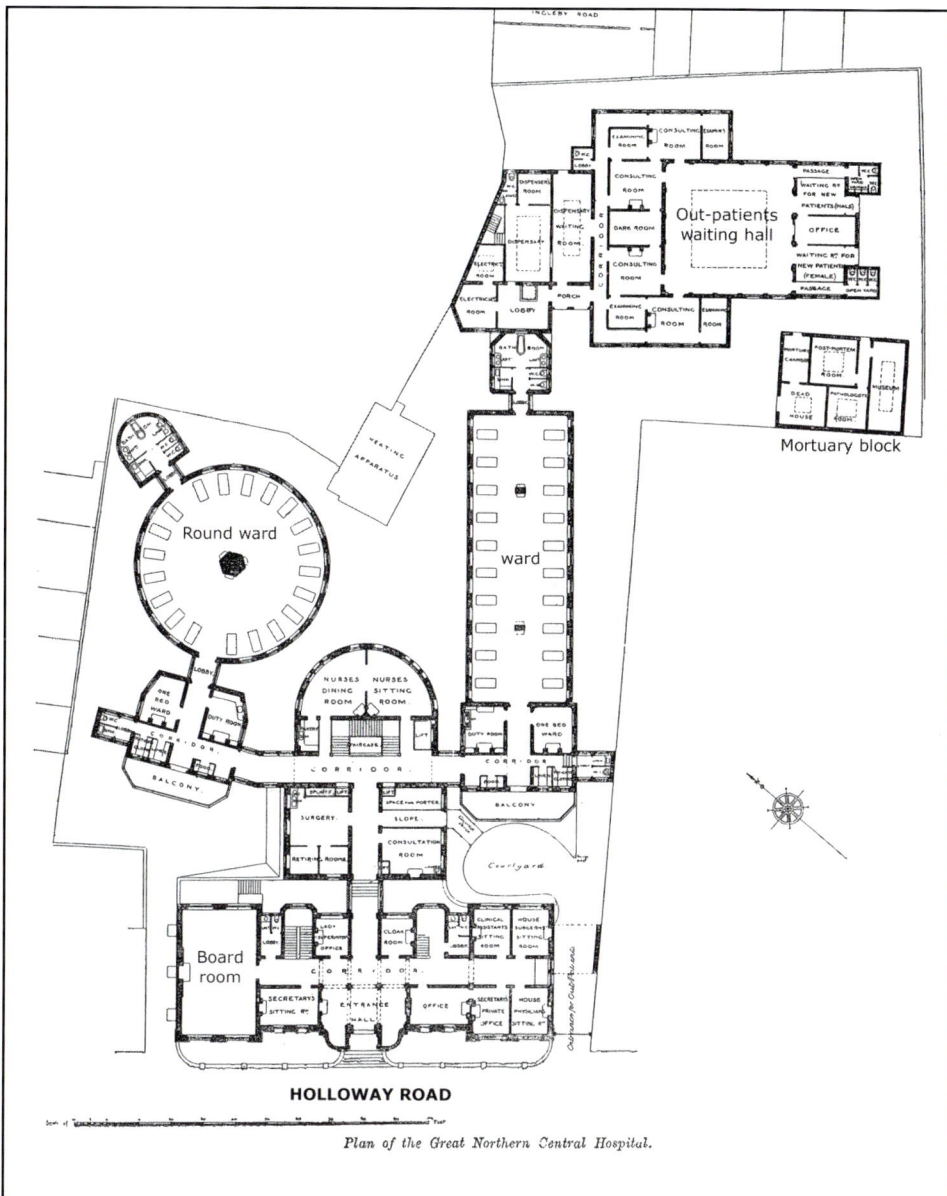

Souvenir Programme.
Courtesy the Royal Northern Hospital Archives, Whittington Hospital

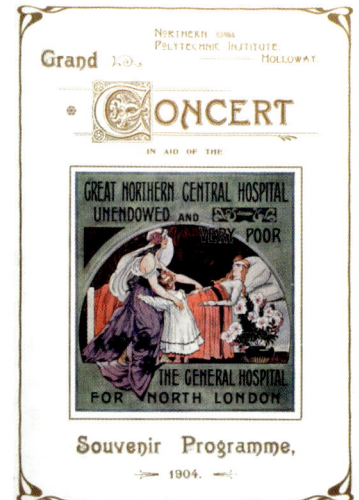

Ground floor plan of new building. The Builder *25 December 1886.*
Courtesy of the London Metropolitan Archives, The Corporation of London

By the end of 1886 building operations had commenced, and over £10,000 was raised. Because of limited funds, it was only possible to erect one block of wards containing sixty beds, the out-patient department, and part of the administration block. In 1888, through fund-raising and a large bequest of £5,000 from a Mr Henry Quinn, the hospital development had reached near completion.

There was now room for 68 patients but the plans eventually provided for 150 and patients were admitted for the first time to the new hospital on 16 April 1888. For three days previously, the buildings were open to the inspection by the general public, and were visited by nearly 6,000 people.

The opening ceremony was postponed by the death of King Frederick III of Germany. The Prince and Princess of Wales, who later became King Edward VII and Queen Alexandra, officially opened the hospital on 17 July 1888.

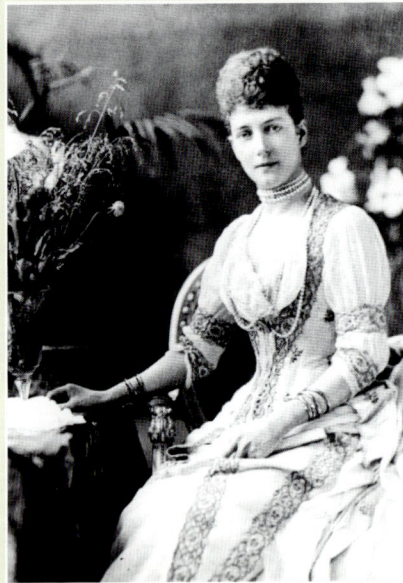

Alexandra Princess of Wales 1889

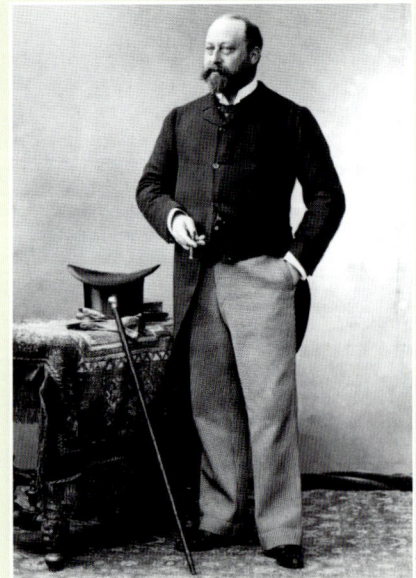

The Royal Archives © 2004
Her Majesty Queen Elizabeth II

Albert Edward Prince of Wales c.1888

Early in 1894 the hospital building was completed. The new wing consisted of the front block on Holloway Road, and the circular block of three wards with accommodation for 65 patients. On the first floor of the Holloway Road block, there were rooms for 19 paying patients. The total number of beds was now raised to over 150. Initially, because of financial constraints, it was only possible to use the top circular ward.

The new wing became known as the Albert Victor Wing, as a memorial to the Duke of Clarence who had become President of the hospital in January 1889. The Duke of Clarence was the brother of the future King George V.

From the *Lancet* correspondent's account when the new buildings were shown to visitors for the first time by the architects, Mr K Young and Mr Henry Hall in February 1888

'*…the hospital consists of three rectangular wards, (twenty beds in each) one above another in a building of three storeys, with a block for administrative purposes and separate buildings for the out-patients and mortuary chambers. It is also in contemplation to erect a block containing three circular block wards (twenty beds in each) and provision is also to be made for the reception of 24 paying patients.*

The outpatients department has been designed to secure at once, the greatest amount of comfort to the patients during their long hours of waiting…

It is intended that the institution shall be open to medical practitioners in the neighbourhood and it may be possible to add to its usefulness by becoming an important postgraduate teaching centre for the north of London.'

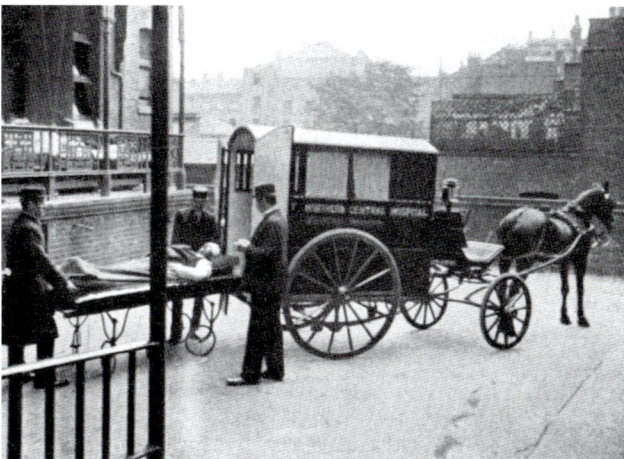

The old horse ambulance brings a casualty into hospital. The ambulance was in use from 1905–1918.
Image courtesy The Royal Northern Hospital 1856–1956 *Eric CO Jewesbury*

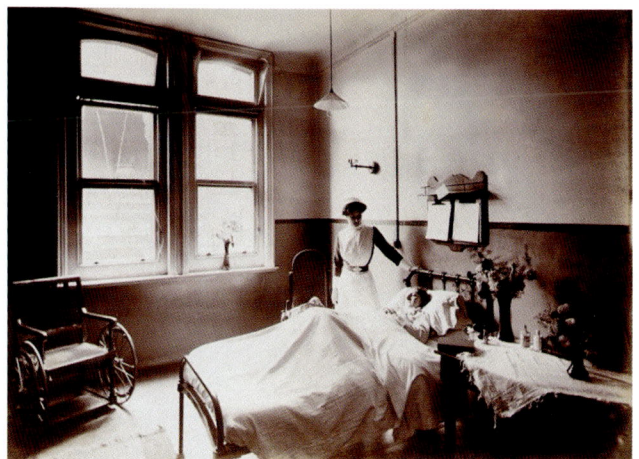

Ward for paying patients, c.1912.
Image courtesy The Wellcome Library, London

The Great Northern Central Hospital, Holloway Road c.1912

7

Selection of silver gelatin photographs from an album in the Wellcome library collection.

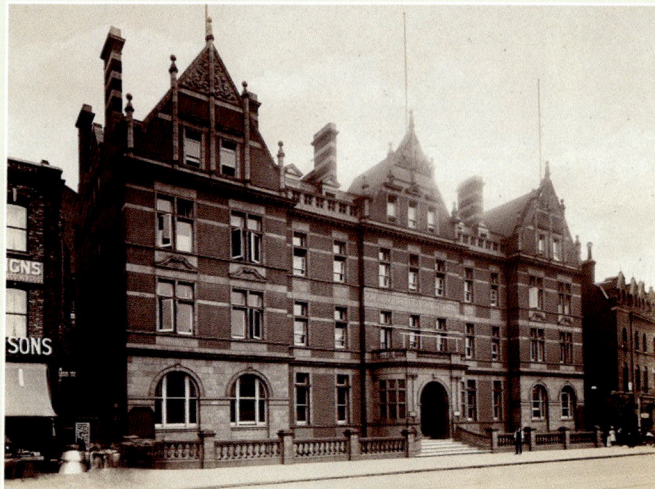

Front View of the Hospital

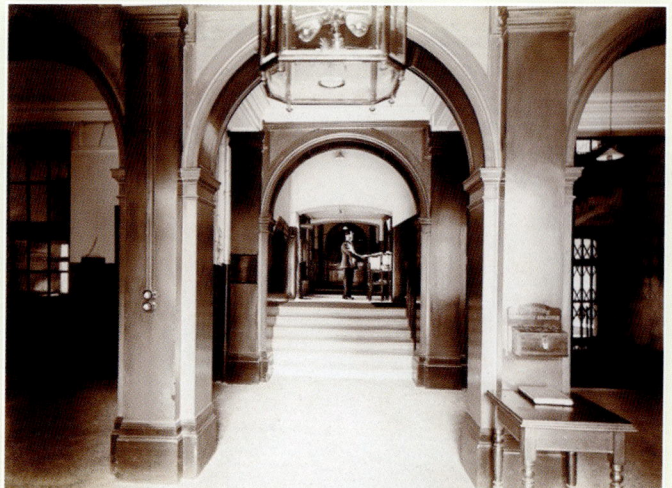

Main entrance hall

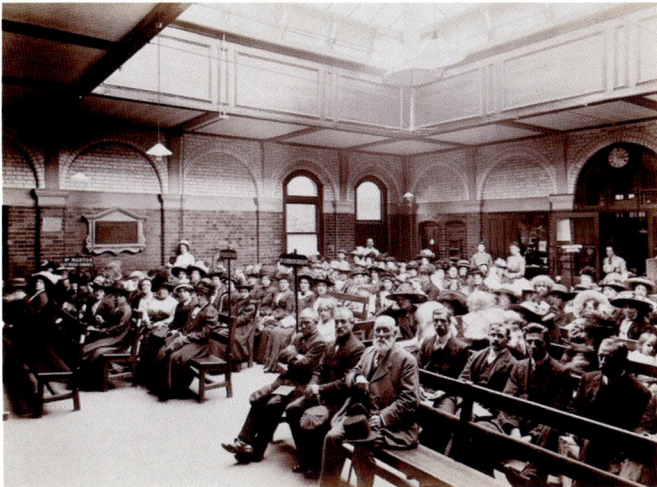

*The out-patients
waiting room*

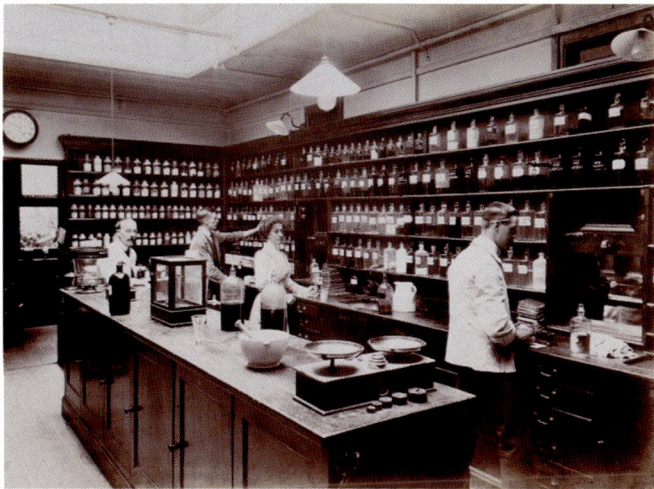

The pharmacy

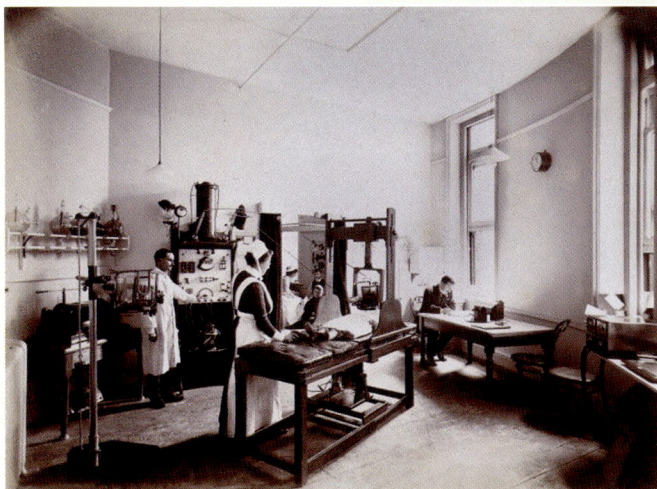

*Patients and staff in
the X-Ray department*

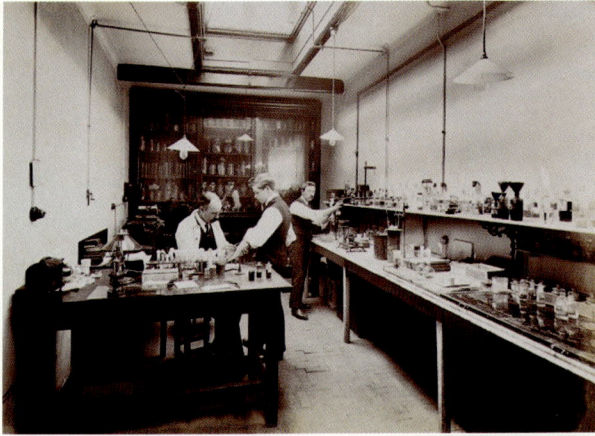

The pathology department

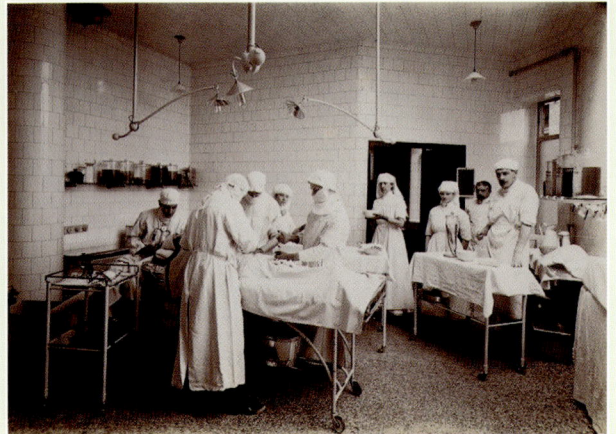

The operating theatre in use

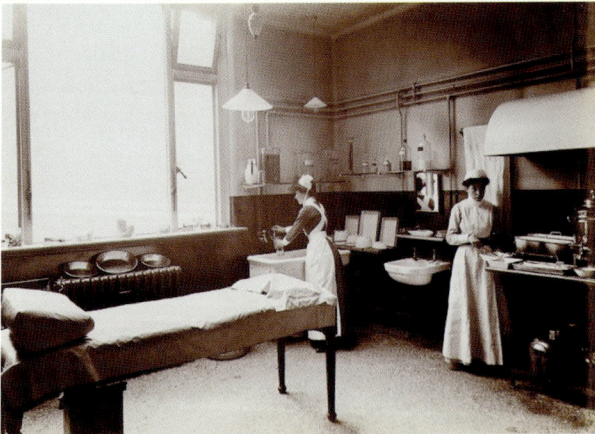

Nurses at work in the surgery

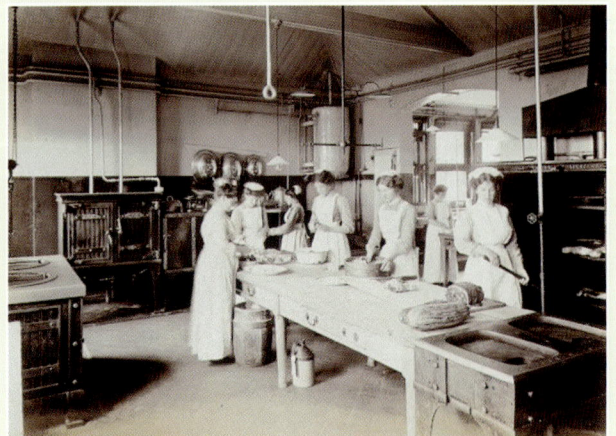

Nurses working in the kitchen

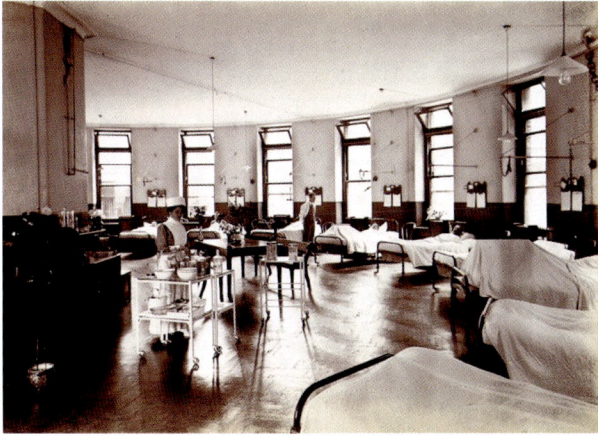

Richard Cloudesley Ward –
right section of one of the circular wards

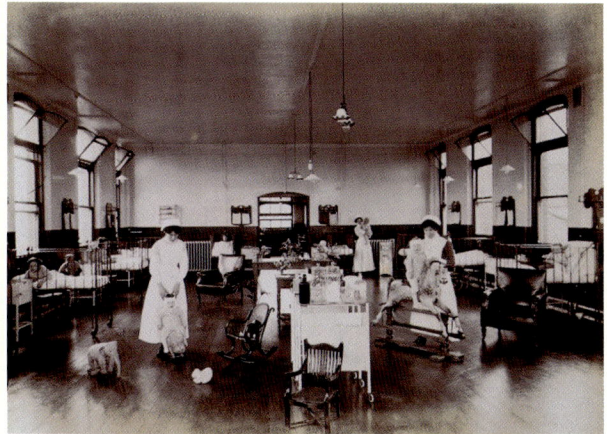

The Annie Zunz ward for children

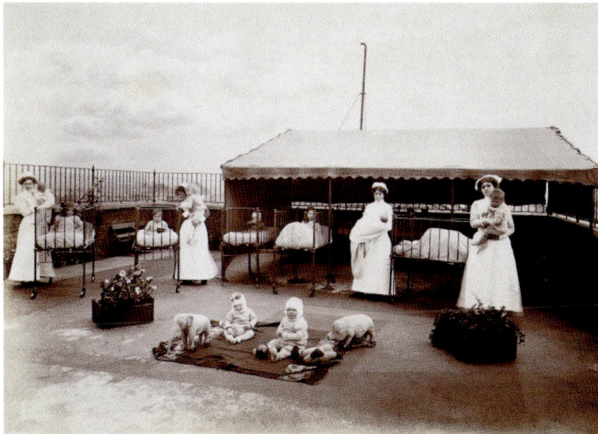

Roof garden to the Annie Zunz ward for children

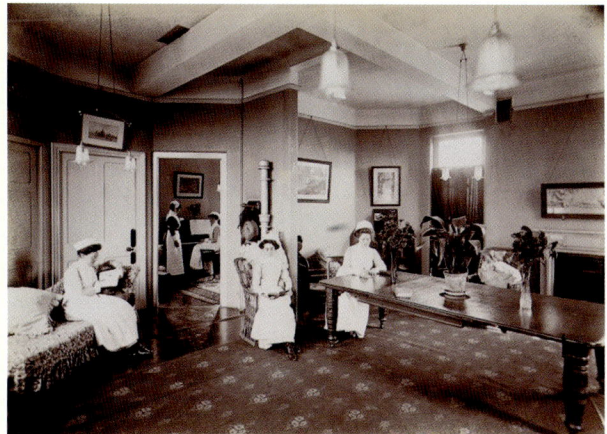

Nursing staff in the common room

Images courtesy The Wellcome Library, London

Royal Assent 1921

8

A meeting of the Management Committee 4 December 1919 unanimously agreed:

> *'That the Annual Council of the Governors be recommended to authorise steps being taken to alter the name of the hospital (Great Northern Central Hospital) to The Royal Northern Hospital, such action involving application to HM The King, to the Privy Council...'*

Moves were delayed until after amalgamation with the Royal Chest Hospital in September 1921.

The following is an extract from a letter dated 22 November 1921, from the Home Office to Lord Northampton, President of the Hospital.

> *'I have the honour by direction of the Secretary of State to inform your Lordship that he has laid before the King, [George V] your application of the 11th ultimo for permission to use the prefix 'Royal' in the title of the Great Northern Central Hospital, and that His Majesty has been graciously pleased to command that the Hospital shall henceforth be known as the Royal Northern Hospital.'*

From that day the hospital assumed its 'Royal' title. A Supplemental Charter recorded the change of name granted 21 June 1924.

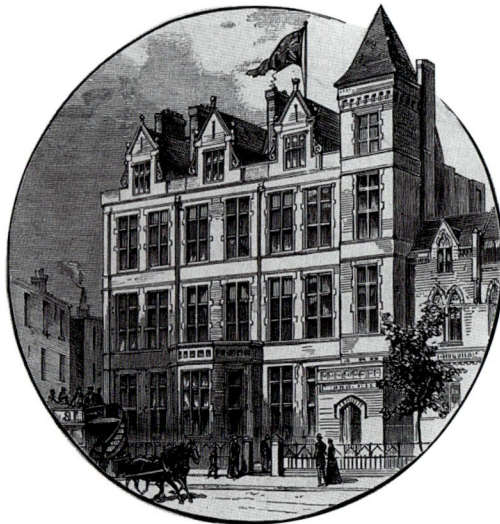

The Royal Chest Hospital, c.1885.
Courtesy The Wellcome Library, London

Annual Report 1932

9

The Annual Report for 1932 included the Royal Northern Hospital, Holloway Road; the Royal Chest Hospital, City Road; the Grovelands Hospital of Recovery, Southgate; the Reckitt Convalescent Home, Clacton-on-Sea and the Maternity Nursing Association, Camden Road.

ROYAL NORTHERN
GROUP OF
HOSPITALS

ROYAL NORTHERN HOSPITAL

ST. DAVID'S WING
(for Private Patients)

ROYAL CHEST HOSPITAL

ANNUAL REPORT
1932

GROVELANDS HOSPITAL (Recovery)   RECKITT CONVALESCENT HOME   MATERNITY NURSING ASSOCIATION

ANNUAL REPORT
OF THE
Royal Northern Hospital
HOLLOWAY ROAD, N.7,
St. David's Wing for Private Patients
MANOR GARDENS, N.7,
The Royal Chest Hospital
CITY ROAD, E.C.1,
Grovelands Hospital (Recovery Branch)
OLD SOUTHGATE, N.14,
The Reckitt Convalescent Home
CLACTON-ON-SEA,
AND
Maternity Nursing Association,
63, MYDDELTON SQUARE, E.C.1, AND 235, CAMDEN ROAD, N.7.
FOR
The Year ending 31st December, 1932.

THE LARGEST GENERAL HOSPITAL IN NORTH LONDON WITH SEPARATE DEPARTMENTS FOR SPECIAL FORMS OF DISEASE.

ESTABLISHED AT KING'S CROSS, JUNE 30TH, 1856,
As THE GREAT NORTHERN HOSPITAL.
AMALGAMATED WITH THE "CENTRAL HOSPITAL FOR NORTH LONDON," 1834.
INCORPORATED BY ROYAL CHARTER, DATED 26TH OCTOBER, 1900.
"THE ROYAL CHEST HOSPITAL," AMALGAMATED, 1921.
SUPPLEMENTAL CHARTER GRANTED 21ST JUNE, 1924, CHANGING THE NAME FROM THE
GREAT NORTHERN CENTRAL HOSPITAL TO THE ROYAL NORTHERN HOSPITAL.
MATERNITY NURSING ASSOCIATION AMALGAMATED, 1930.
ST. DAVID'S WING FOR PRIVATE PATIENTS BUILT AND OPENED 1931.

NO LETTERS OF RECOMMENDATION ARE NECESSARY.
The necessitous poor are treated free of all charges.
Contributions towards maintenance are received from patients able to afford it.
CASES OF EMERGENCY ARE RECEIVED AT ANY HOUR OF THE DAY OR NIGHT.
TELEPHONES:
Hospital—Archway 2211 (6 lines).   Royal Chest Hospital—Clerkenwell 1218.
St. David's Wing—Archway 2211 Ext. 40. Maternity Nursing Assoc. Clo. 6395 North 5487.
Grovelands Hospital—Palmer's Green 3636.   Convalescent Home—Clacton 105.

THE LARGEST HOSPITAL SERVICE IN NORTH LONDON

which, seventy-six years ago, occupied one room in the York Road, now consists of a group of four Hospitals with four hundred and sixty-six beds. The demands on its services are still increasing, as is shown by the comparative figures below.

	1913	1932
In-Patients	2,330	5,937
Out-Patient Attendances	87,000	325,776
Cost of Annual Maintenance	£21,382	£108,244
	(Pre-war prices)	

The Hospital possesses thirty special departments which include a Maternity Department. There is also a Private Wing for paying patients.

There is a debt of £134,867
Your help, and the help of your friends is earnestly solicited

The Group consists of:—
ROYAL NORTHERN HOSPITAL, Holloway, N.7
ST. DAVID'S WING (for private patients), Manor Gardens, N.7
ROYAL CHEST HOSPITAL, City Road, E.C.1
GROVELANDS HOSPITAL (Recovery), Southgate, N.14
RECKITT CONVALESCENT HOME, Clacton-on-Sea
MATERNITY NURSING ASSOCIATION,
Myddelton Square, E.C.1 and 235, Camden Road, N.7
(for District Midwifery work with Ante-Natal and Infant Welfare Clinics).

Donations and subscriptions should be sent to the Secretary (Gilbert G. Panter),
Royal Northern Hospital, Holloway, N.7

The Group serves over a MILLION people in an area of seventy square miles.

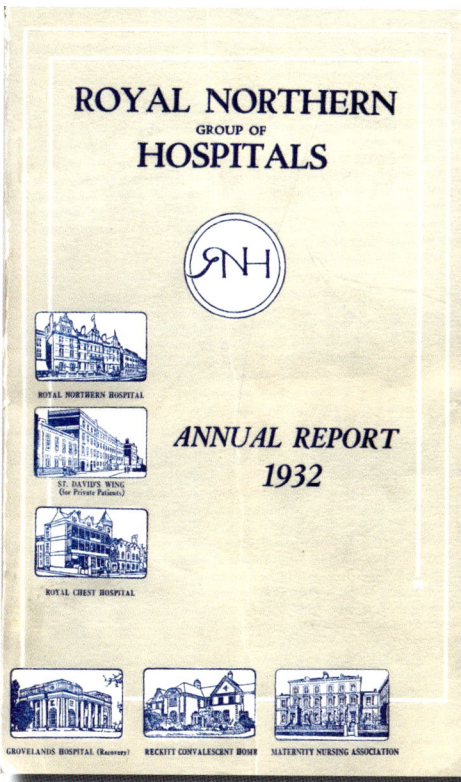

Extracts from the Annual Report – 1932.
Courtesy the Royal Northern Hospital Archives, Whittington Hospital

St David's Wing

10

In 1928, Sir Howell Williams, a very wealthy businessman and benefactor to the hospital, came forward with a proposal; this was the building of a Private Pay-beds Block adjacent to the main hospital. He offered to contribute £35,000 for the construction of the Block, if a similar sum could be raised to meet the urgent needs of the hospital. This munificent offer stimulated others to respond generously which included the King's Fund and at a Festival Dinner, over £14,000 was raised. Generous donors rose to the challenge and the whole of the crucial £35,000 was raised by the end of the year and plans for the building were prepared.

In 1929 two old houses in Manor Gardens were demolished and the new private block, to be known as St David's Wing, began to

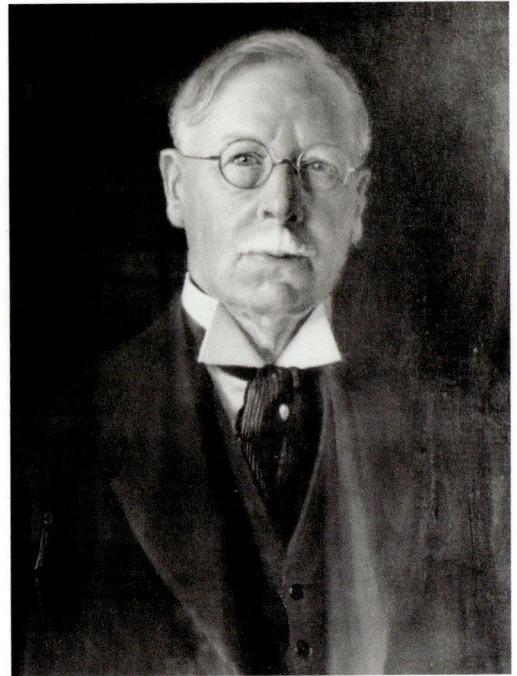

Portrait of Sir Howell J Williams JP, c.1935 by W R Brealey ROI
Courtesy the Royal Northern Hospital Archives, Whittington Hospital

take shape adjoining the old Nurses' Home. By 1931 the first section was completed, and the Wing contained fifty-five single and five double bedrooms, arranged on three floors with reception rooms and consulting rooms on the ground floor. Two operating theatres and a special kitchen were added. The bedrooms were nicely furnished and fitted with running hot and cold water. Each room had a telephone, wireless head-phones and signalling lamps for the attention of nurses. The floors were named Ifor, Trevor and Meyrick after Sir Howell Williams' three sons.

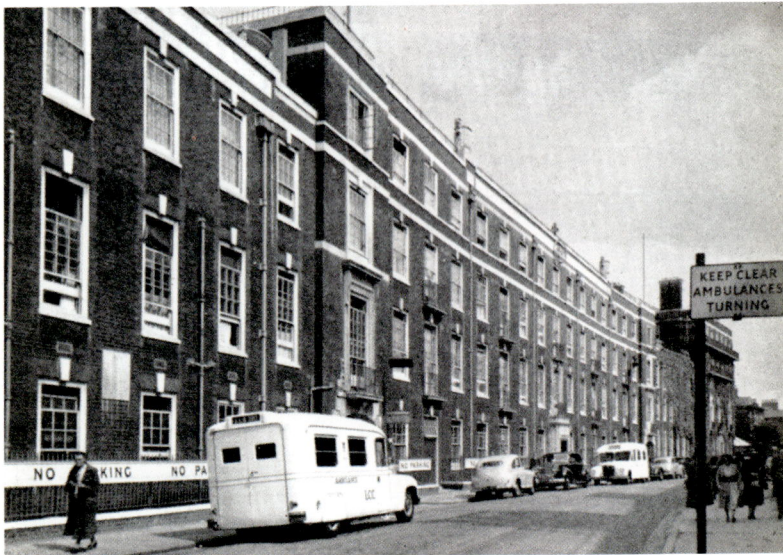

St David's Wing, Manor Gardens – 1950s
Courtesy The Royal Northern Hospital 1856–1956. Eric CO Jewesbury

One son, Captain Ifor Williams, was killed in action 9 October 1918, and the Captain Ifor Williams Ward in the main hospital was named in his memory.

The private Wing was for patients who were unable to afford full professional and nursing home fees and was intended for those patients requiring a short stay for medical or surgical treatment. The original charge for rooms was from five to ten guineas per week. Patients were entitled to put themselves under the care of any physician or surgeon who was on the senior staff of any recognised London hospital.

More private rooms were added, seven of which could be used for maternity cases, and a small labour ward was opened on the second floor. In November 1935 the building was finished; and Sir Howell Williams had contributed altogether £57,000 towards the cost of this project.

St David's Wing was the first of its kind in this country and by 1935 it had gained a high reputation, not only in the district but also throughout London and the Provinces. More than a thousand patients used the Wing each year and it managed to be selfsupporting. Advice was requested from the Hospital Secretary by other hospitals how to build and run similar Wings.

In 1936 Sir Howell Williams provided £5,000 towards the construction of a new Nurses' Home. In 1937 he gave £32,000 towards the conversion of the existing Nurses' Home into a Private Maternity Section and £20,000 for provision of a Home for St David's Wing Nurses. In all, Sir Howell Williams had contributed £158,000 (equivalent of about £6,300,000 to-day) to the Royal Northern Hospital and was the hospital's greatest benefactor. It was said of him, 'He possessed his wealth; he never allowed it to possess him.' He represented South Islington for 27 consecutive years on the London County Council, becoming Deputy Chairman. Sir Howell died in his eightieth year in August 1939.

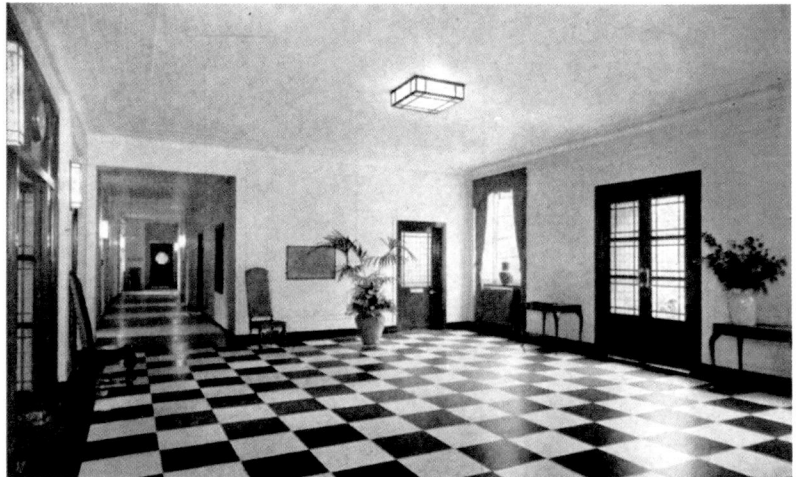

Entrance hall of St David's Wing – 1950s.

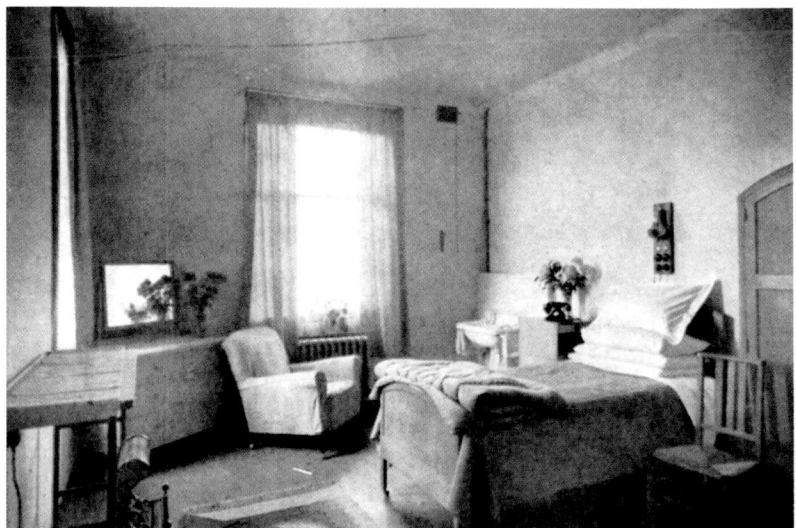

One of the bedrooms – 1950s.

Images courtesy The Royal Northern Hospital 1856–1956. *Eric CO Jewesbury*

The Beecham Laboratories – 1937

11

Through the generosity of Messrs. Beechams Pills Ltd, and the instrumentality of Mr Phillip Hill, Chairman of the company, the Board are very glad to report that a further step has been taken in adding to the facilities already available for scientific investigation into the cause of disease and its diagnosis. The Company gave the handsome sum of £14,200 following which a building carefully planned for its special purpose, was completed and graciously opened by HRH The Duchess of Gloucester on October 26th (1937) Mr Phillip Hill having previously laid the foundation stone December 8th 1936. The most modern accommodation and equipment for Pathological, Bacteriological, Biochemical and Pharmaceutical investigations have been provided. Mr Phillip Hill, at the opening ceremony, generously intimated that his company would also provide £1000 per annum towards additional cost of maintaining this Section. The Board desire publicly to record their deep gratitude for this valued gift which has still further enhanced the efficacy of the services which the Hospital is able to offer to the Sick.

The Beecham Laboratory Annual Report 1937. Royal Northern Group of Hopitals.

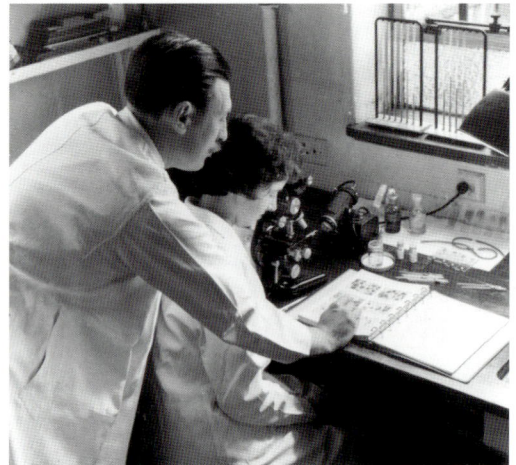

Mr Frank Cain, chief laboratory technician, teaching Ann Baird (a trainee), cell morphology using the Sandoz Atlas.

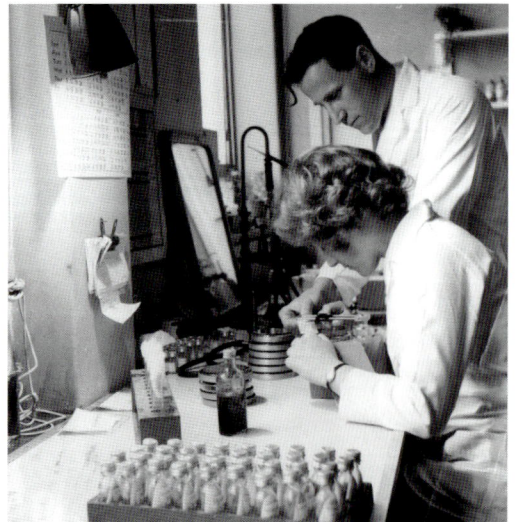

Mr Tony Hadley, senior laboratory technician, demonstrating to a trainee the morphology of bacterial colonies. Photographs c.1970.

Images courtesy the Royal Northern Hospital Archives, Whittington Hospital

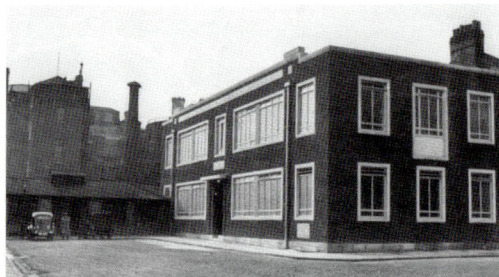

The Beecham Laboratory, purpose built pathology department

Dr Beatrix Wonke OBE MD FRCPath
A personal account

On the first of May 1977, I started in my new post as Consultant Clinical Haematologist at the Royal Northern Hospital.

I was the first generation of clinical haematologists with laboratory and clinical responsibilities. The department of haematology occupied the ground floor of the Beecham Laboratory. The haematology laboratory consisted of a large room with work-benches, microscopes, test tubes and minimal automation; next to it was the blood transfusion room, then Miss Ellis's room (chief laboratory technician) with my room being shared with the secretary. We also had a large room which was occupied by a trainee haematologist and visiting foreign doctors.

The location of the Beecham Laboratory was such that my consultant colleagues and general practitioners had to pass it from the car park to the main building. This gave them the opportunity to visit us and discuss diagnostic problems, or to bring in blood samples for analysis. The Royal Northern Hospital was memorable for this close collegial environment.

The departments of bacteriology, biochemistry and histopathology were very close which helped to solve diagnostic conundrums quickly.

Shortly after my arrival we started modernising the laboratory by investing in the purchase of a semi-automated Coulter counter. This allowed a larger input of blood samples to be analysed. This could be done more quickly than the manual method.

Over the years I gained the confidence of my clinical colleagues and the general practitioners. My clinical practice grew considerably, and this required hospital beds and the appointment of junior trainee haematologists. Those posts were for one year, so the turnover in junior staff was considerable.

Whilst working at the Royal Northern Hospital I became aware of thalassaemia, a little known condition in the United Kingdom. It occurs in the immigrant population from the Mediterranean, Indian sub-continent, the Middle East and Far East. Thalassaemia is an inherited severe blood disorder; children can only survive with life-long blood transfusions. The technical staff in my laboratory became experts in diagnosing this condition, and with their help, our research activities reached international levels.

Clinical Research Fellows came to work with us from Italy, Cyprus, Iran and Iraq. As our reputation grew in the management of thalassaemia, our pool of foreign patients also

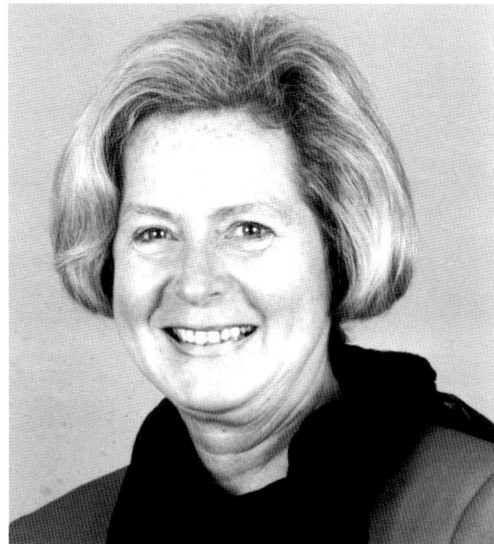

Dr Beatrix Wonke OBE MD FRCPath.
Photograph courtesy Dr Beatrix Wonke

increased with its many problem cases to be solved. This contributed to the post-graduate teaching programme of the hospital under Dr Geraint James' directorship.

Training United Kingdom and visiting doctors for the MRCP (Membership of the Royal College of Physicians) examination, was an important part of the hospital work in which all my colleagues contributed. The milieu was intimate, warm-hearted, humorous and most of all patient orientated.

Unfortunately the National Health Service started to change by the 1980s and the political dictum was that of reduction of expenditure, hospital closures, and rationalisation of resources. The sad consequence was the closure of the Royal Northern Hospital. We all moved to the Whittington Hospital. Life took on a new meaning and a new era started, but we never forgot the days in the Royal Northern Hospital.

Dr Roger Bird PhD C.Chem. FRSC Consultant Clinical Biochemist Head of the Biochemistry Department 1960–1990

A personal account

In 1946 Dr Raymond Greene DM FRCP (1901–1982) was appointed consultant physician to the Royal Northern Hospital; his brother was Graham Greene the celebrated author. The highlight of Dr Greene's mountaineering career came with his membership of the 1933 Everest Expedition. He was the senior doctor for that mission and became an expert on frostbite. During World War II he was medical officer to intelligence agents that were being sent to France. On Coronation Day in 1953, it was

Dr Greene who announced on the BBC that Hillary and Tenzing had climbed Everest.

Dr Greene was one of the first clinicians to recognise the importance of endocrinology in medicine and edited an early textbook on the subject; *The Practice of Clinical Endocrinology* published in 1948. I knew him well, as I worked with him at New End Hospital, Hampstead and later at the Royal Northern Hospital. At the inauguration of the National Health Service he had been appointed consultant physician to the Royal Northern Hospital and the thyroid clinic at New End Hospital. Under his guidance the thyroid clinic expanded to cover the whole of endocrinology. It was at the New End Hospital that I became interested in endocrine biochemistry and it was there that I published an early method for the estimation of protein bound iodine, a test for thyroid dysfunction.

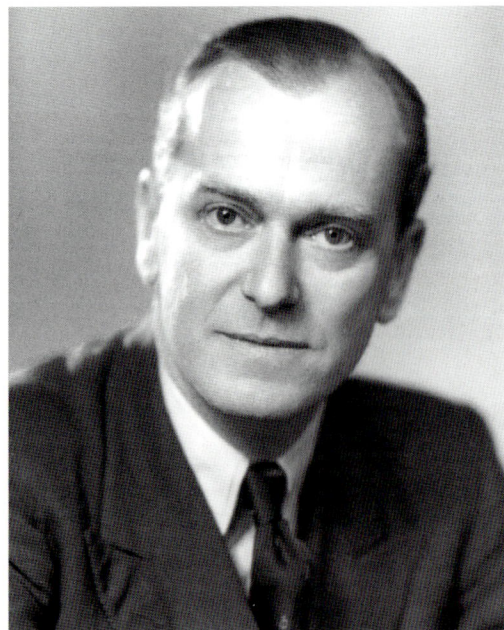

Dr Raymond Greene DM FRCP. Elliott & Fry 1952. Courtesy of the National Portrait Gallery London

When I was appointed to the Royal Northern Hospital in 1960, few general hospitals were able to provide protein bound iodine as a test for thyroid disease. The method was difficult and time consuming, taking a full working day to complete. Results had to be interpreted with care and needed experience of the problems involved. We were frequently asked to help other hospitals requiring this test. Today specific thyroid hormone investigations are requested in large numbers and using modern analytical systems results can be obtained within thirty minutes. How times have changed.

Following the retirement of Dr Raymond Greene in 1966, Dr Bill Havard MD FRCP was appointed consultant physician to the Royal Northern Hospital and the special interest in endocrinology continued. Another major achievement was the creation of the clinical pharmacology unit in 1975–1990. This was the first co-operative venture between the pharmaceutical industry and the NHS. It was subsidised by Pfizer Limited and was under the joint directorship of Dr Bill Havard physician and Dr Michael East, clinical research director of Pfizer Limited.

The staff consisted of a senior registrar, two senior house officers, a biochemist and a ward sister. The clinical pharmacology unit was situated on the top floor of St David's Wing where a new laboratory was designed and fully equipped. I recall how the presence of this unit provided new opportunities for the collaboration between my department and the unit both for research and staff training. Dr Anoja Fernando was one of a number of overseas post-graduate doctors working in the unit. On returning to Sri Lanka she became Professor of Pharmacology and later Dean of the Medical School.

At the same time new equipment was given to the biochemistry department. This extended the research capabilities of the laboratory and I well remember working with Dr Geraint James and his team in a study of the biochemistry of sarcoidosis.

During the last few years our biochemistry department worked jointly with the biochemistry department of the Whittington Hospital and achieved a successful merger on the Whittington Hospital site when the laboratories at the Royal Northern Hospital finally closed.

The Royal Northern Hospital achieved much in its long existence and its staff had a great ethos of working together as a team. Everyone who worked at the hospital whom I have since met have happy memories of their time spent working there.

I can think of no better way of concluding than to reiterate the words of Dr Geraint James 'What a pity it had to end!'

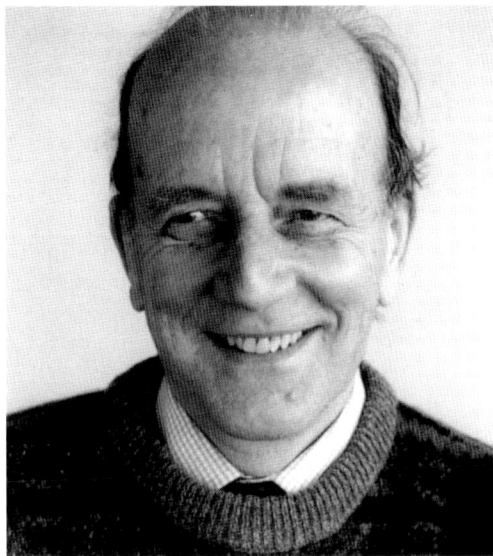

Dr Roger Bird PhD C.Chem. FRSC.

Photograph courtesy Dr Roger Bird

Sir Lancelot Barrington-Ward KCVO ChM FRCS (1884-1953)

12

Lancelot Barrington-Ward was born at Worcester on 4 July 1884, to Mark and Caroline Barrington-Ward; his father Canon Mark Barrington-Ward was an Inspector of Schools. They had five sons who all distinguished themselves; one, Robert, became editor of The Times.

Lancelot Barrington-Ward entered Worcester College Oxford with a classical exhibition. He received his medical training at Edinburgh University and qualified with honours in 1908. In the same year he was captain of the University Rugby XV and represented England in four internationals. He obtained the Edinburgh FRCS in 1910 and the English FRCS in 1912. From Edinburgh he obtained the ChM (Master of Surgery) with honours in 1913. In 1914 he was appointed surgeon to the Great Northern Hospital, which was later to be renamed the Royal Northern Hospital.

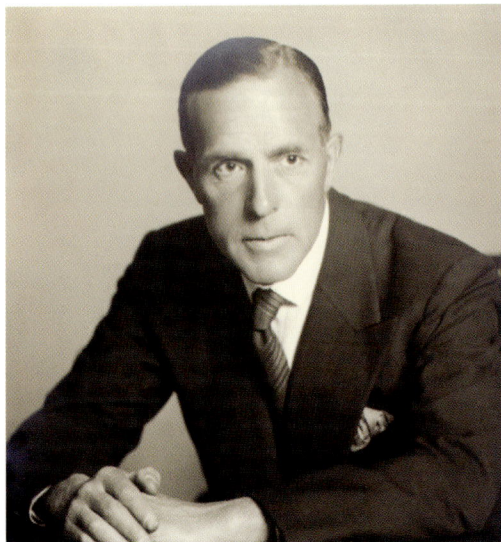

Sir Lancelot Barrington-Ward. Photograph c.1950s.

Courtesy Dr Breda Barrington-Ward

Lancelot Barrington-Ward was appointed house surgeon to the Hospital for Sick Children, Great Ormond Street in 1910, and was appointed assistant surgeon in 1914. He married Dorothy Miles in 1917, and they had three daughters. His wife Dorothy was very involved with the Peter Pan League. This charity was set up as a children's club following J M Barrie's copyright gift to the hospital in 1929 and helped to raise money through the efforts of children of the wealthy. Dorothy was secretary from its establishment in 1930, until her premature death in 1935. Lancelot Barrington-Ward later married Catherine Reuter, and they had a son, Dr Edward Barrington-Ward who graduated from Cambridge and St Bartholomew's Hospital. He went into general practice in Bury St Edmunds, Suffolk and was one of the founder members of St Nicholas Hospice there, before moving North to take up the post of Medical Director of the Highland Hospice in Inverness. He died in July 1998 at the early age of fifty-five.

Whilst he was still a young man, Barrington-Ward's ability as a surgeon, was widely recognised. In 1934 he was consulted by Albert, Duke of York (the future King George VI), on whom he operated for a very severe infection of his hand. The infection began to spread up the forearm and a second operation was performed. Fortunately this potentially life-threatening infection began to subside and the patient, the

Duke of York, recovered. This was before the sulphonamides became available in England, in 1936.

Lancelot Barrington-Ward was created KCVO in 1935, and subsequently became Surgeon to the Household of King George VI and later, Extra Surgeon to the Household of Queen Elizabeth II. One of his most notable fields was in was the surgery of the stomach and gall-bladder, but it was for his expertise in children's surgery that he was best known. He was appointed Hunterian Professor at the Royal College of Surgeons, England in 1952. He was author of the textbook *Abdominal Surgery of Children* and was editor of two editions of *Royal Northern Operative Surgery*.

'His patience and gentleness with patients were outstanding, and unlike some of his predecessors, he behaved with punctilious courtesy in the operating theatre. The Royal Northern Hospital has numbered many distinguished surgeons on its staff but Sir Lancelot Barrington-Ward will long be remembered not only for his professional ability but also for his loyalty and his hospital obligations'.

Courtesy The Royal Northern Hospital 1856–1956 *Eric CO Jewesbury.*

Sir Lancelot Barrington-Ward retired from the post of Senior Surgeon to the hospital in 1952, and sadly died from cancer in November 1953, aged sixty-nine.

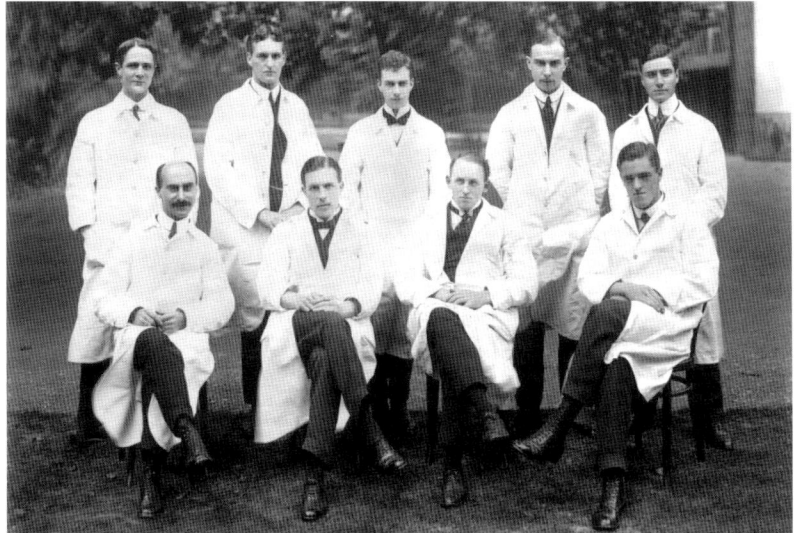

T.S.LUKIS H.P.   D.D.RITCHIE H.S.   J.INKSTER A.C.M.   T.T.HIGGINS H.S.   C.E.SHATTOCK H.S.

D.NABARRO PATHOLOGIST   L.E.BARRINGTON WARD R.M.O.   R.R.ARMSTRONG M.R.   H.H.SAMPSON C.M.O.

Group of Residents c.1913 – Great Ormond Street Hospital for Sick Children.
Courtesy the Museum and Archive Service, Great Ormond Street Hospital for Children NHS Trust

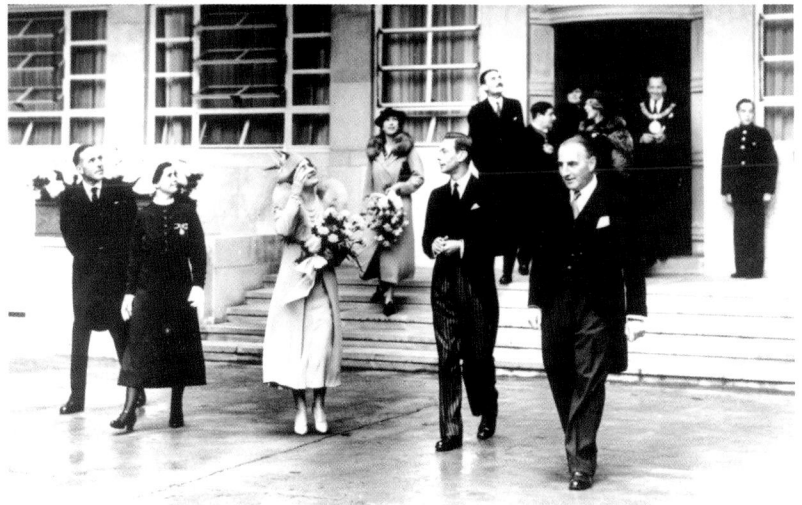

Great Ormond Street Hospital for Sick Children. 18 October 1938.
A visit of HM Queen Elizabeth (the late Queen Mother) and the late King George VI, to view the new wards, operating theatres and laboratories of the Southwood Wing. Behind Queen Elizabeth is Princess Mary, who was Princess Royal, the eldest daughter of King George V. To the extreme left are Sir Lancelot Barrington-Ward and the Matron, Miss Dorothy Lane.
Courtesy the Daily Sketch and Dr Breda Barrington-Ward

Lord Horder of Ashford GCVO DCL MD FRCP (1871–1955)

13

Thomas Jeeves Horder was born on 7 January 1871 in Shaftesbury, Dorset. His father was Albert Horder, a businessman in Swindon. Young Thomas Horder was educated at Swindon High School, and later became a student at St Bartholomew's Hospital, where he was an outstanding undergraduate student, winning many scholarships. He took the final MB degree with first class honours and Gold Medals in 1896. His first hospital appointment was as house physician to Dr Samuel Gee (1839–1911), one of the outstanding teachers and personalities of the hospital at that time.

In 1912 Dr Horder was appointed Assistant Physician to St Bartholomew's Hospital.

Undoubtedly, the greatest physician to be associated with the Royal Northern Hospital was Lord Horder. He was appointed to the honorary staff in 1899 and took an active part in the medical administrative affairs of the hospital. Reluctantly, in April 1913, he sent his resignation to the Management Committee of the Great Northern Hospital; he was, however, persuaded to stay on for a further year. In 1933 he was elected Consultant Physician to the now Royal Northern Hospital. He also had the honour of being Orator to the Medical Society of London.

As a young physician he was called into consultation by the medical advisors to King Edward VII. They found that the King had glycosuria but above the bed of his patient, Dr Horder observed a number of bottles of patent medicines, among them a popular remedy used to treat rheumatism. He knew that these medicines contained salicylates. After the King had stopped taking the patent medicines Dr Horder found that the diagnosis of glycosuria was incorrect!

Dr Horder was knighted in 1918, and early in the reign of George VI, he became Physician in Ordinary to the King. In 1933 he was elevated to the peerage as Lord Horder of Ashford. Later he became Extra Physician to Queen Elizabeth II.

His greatest influence as a teacher was perhaps the example he set at the bedside of the patient, in his adherence to the classical routine of a thorough clinical examination. His retentive memory and heightened capacity to observe, made him a virtuoso in spot diagnosis. However, that was based on the thoroughness with which, over the years, he had trained his powers of observation.

In his farewell lecture at St Bartholomew's Hospital in 1936, he spoke of the three great advances he had witnessed in his time. The first was the integration of morbid anatomy with clinical medicine, the second the development of laboratory methods bringing about the birth of clinical pathology, and the third the arrival of x-rays. Horder might well be called the 'father of clinical pathology'.

Lord Horder died of a coronary thrombosis on 13 August 1955. His death removed the most outstanding clinician of his time, and the personality best known in British medicine, to the general public.

ON DIAGNOSIS

Paraphrasing the well known description of his art attributed to Demosthenes*, it has been said of medicine that 'the most important thing is diagnosis; the next most important thing is diagnosis; and the third most important thing is diagnosis'.

In diagnosis, one physical sign is of more value than many symptoms.

As 'probability is the very guide of life,' so it is the guide of diagnosis. Cæteris paribus†, a common disease is more likely than an uncommon one to be the explanation of any particular set of signs and symptoms. This is a statement, which it would seem absurd to make, if the fact were not so frequently forgotten.

MEDICAL NOTES
by Sir Thomas Horder MD.

Henry Frowde, Oxford University Press 1921

* Demosthenes (384–322BC) was a prominent Greek statesman and orator of ancient Athens.

† All things being equal.

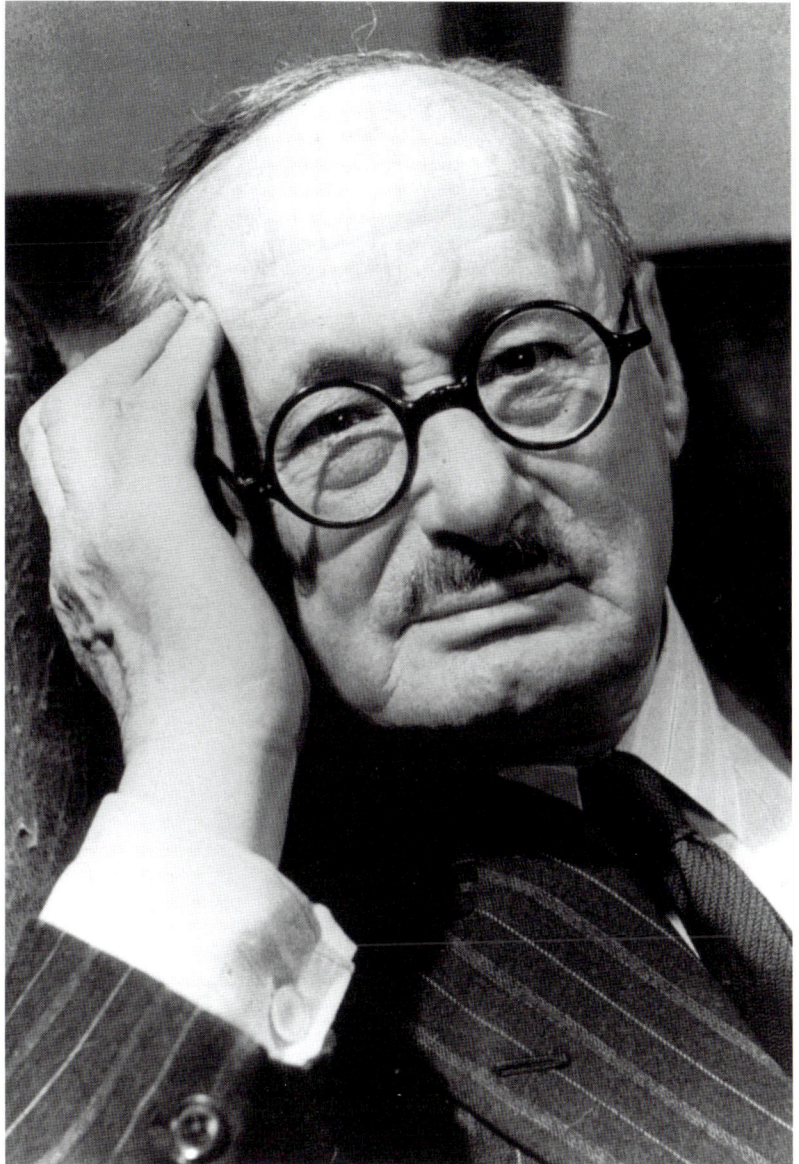

Lord Horder GCVO MD DCL FRCP. Photograph by Douglas Glass 1953
This photograph hung in the old board room in the Royal Northern Hospital.
Courtesy The Sunday Times Portrait Gallery

Henry Hamilton Bailey FRCS (1894-1961)

14

Henry Hamilton Bailey was born on 1 October 1894 at Bishopstoke, Hampshire. His father, Dr James Bailey was a general practitioner. The family eventually moved to Brighton where his father had a busy practice. Unfortunately his mother, Margaret Bailey, suffered from a severe recurrent mental illness and later alcoholism; Bailey's younger sister, May, developed schizophrenia. Because of the family situation young Bailey's early education was spent at a boarding school, St Lawrence College, Ramsgate, where he excelled at swimming.

Hamilton Bailey entered the London Hospital Medical College in 1912, but the First World War interrupted his studies. In August 1914 he volunteered as a dresser for the British Red Cross Society. The Unit was sent to Brussels and shortly after arrival, the Germans occupied the city. One day, Hamilton Bailey was returning from Brussels to Scharbeck Station outside Brussels, where he and his fellow colleagues had been treating allied wounded prisoners of war, on their way to Germany. Because Bailey had no valid papers, he was arrested by the Germans and imprisoned on suspicion as a spy, where his fate was all but sealed. Two other members of his unit were also imprisoned with him on the same charges. Had it not been for the intervention of the American Ambassador, Brand Whitlock, they would all have been executed. The following year, Whitlock's intercession on behalf of Edith Cavell was less successful, she was executed by firing squad 12 October 1915.

Subsequently, repatriation was arranged for the whole Unit. After further adventures including re-arrest and further American intervention they travelled through Germany, then to Denmark, the party finally arriving in Newcastle in October 1914.

In 1915 he was a final year medical student and he volunteered in the Royal Navy as Surgeon Probationer RNVR, and in 1916 qualified as a doctor by taking the Licentiate of the Society of Apothecaries examination. He served in the battleship HMS Iron Duke

Microscopy drawings from Hamilton Bailey's student's notebook 1912.

Courtesy the Royal Northern Hospital Archives, Whittington Hospital

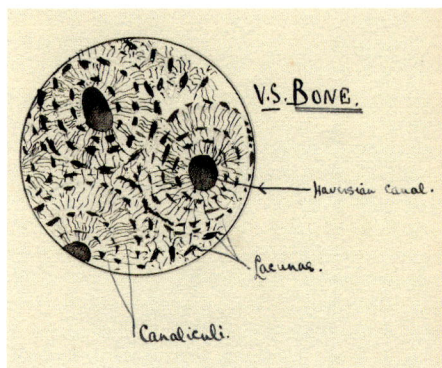

Section of bone

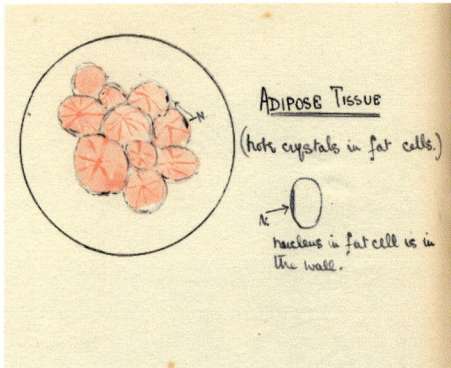

Adipose tissue

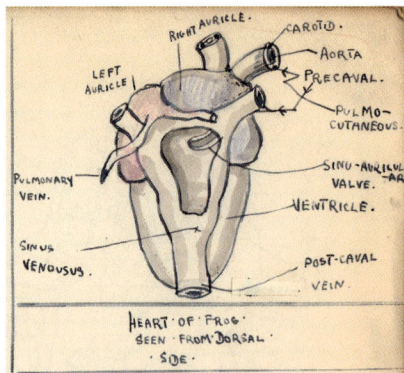

Heart of frog

during the Battle of Jutland and dealt with many casualties. He was promoted to Surgeon Lieutenant RN, and served aboard HMS Inflexible and HMS Monitor.

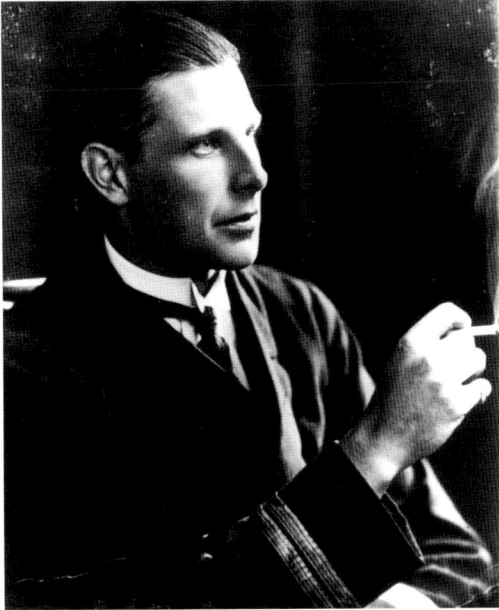

Hamilton Bailey Surgeon Lieutenant RN c.1916.
©Royal London Hospital Archives

Hamilton Bailey obtained the FRCS in 1920, and then held the post of surgical registrar at the London Hospital. He became First Assistant to Sir Hugh Rigby and Sir James Walton in 1923 but did not succeed in joining the honorary staff as Assistant Surgeon when he sought election in 1925. The competition was tough, Hugh Cairns was one of two successful candidates, who went on to become a pioneer neurosurgeon and first Professor of Surgery at the University of Oxford. In 1924 whilst working at the London Hospital, Bailey accidentally injured his left index finger during an emergency operation for peritonitis. This resulted in a severe infection of his hand and arm. Unfortunately he was left with a stiff but useless finger and eventually he had

to submit to an amputation. This almost cut short his surgical career but in the event he resumed operating and fortunately, he found that his skills were unimpaired.

In 1925 he was awarded the Gillson scholarship of the Society of Apothecaries. He applied for the post as assistant surgeon to the Liverpool Royal Infirmary, and was successful. During this period Bailey started work on the production of his first textbook, *Demonstrations of Physical Signs in Clinical Surgery*, which was published in 1927. His idea was to profusely illustrate his textbook, and at the time this was a pioneering concept, but he needed a suitable photographic studio

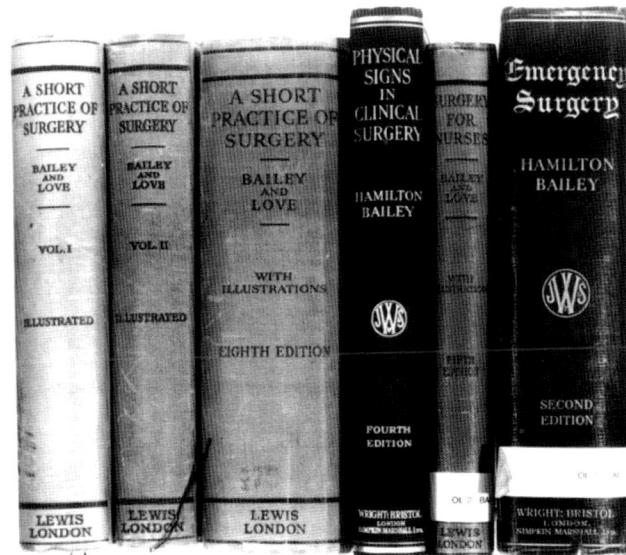

A selection of textbooks written by Hamilton Bailey FRCS and some jointly with RJ McNeill Love MS FRCS.
A Short Practice of Surgery. *Bailey & Love. First published in 1932 in two volumes, subsequently in one volume.*
A Short Practice of Surgery. *Bailey & Love. Eighth edition 1949.*
Physical Signs in Clinical Surgery. *Hamilton Bailey. Fourth edition 1933, first published 1927.*
Surgery for Nurses. *Bailey & Love. Fifth edition 1942, first published 1933.*
Emergency Surgery. *Hamilton Bailey. Second edition 1936, first published 1930.*
©Royal London Hospital Archives.

to carry out this work. He found one, which was managed by a pretty young photographer, Veta Gillender, whom he married in 1926. She developed an expertise in medical photography which included the use of colour photography (rare in medical books of the 1930s and 1940s). Her kindness and skill in putting her subjects at ease, contributed significantly to the success of the books.

In 1925, there was a further move from Liverpool to Birmingham to the Dudley Road Hospital, where he gained considerable experience in emergency surgery. He had ninety beds of his own and no house surgeon to help him and he performed three thousand five hundred operations in four years. During his next move to the Bruce Wills Hospital, Bristol in 1930, the first edition of his book *Emergency Surgery* was published. Finally, in 1930 Hamilton Bailey returned to London

on his appointment to the staff of the Royal Northern Hospital as consultant surgeon urologist. In 1940 the first edition of his book *The Surgery of Modern Warfare* was published and was adopted by the Royal Army Medical Services.

In 1947, he was awarded a Hunterian Professorship at the Royal College of Surgeons of England and in the same year was elected a Fellow of the Royal Society of Edinburgh. Bailey held a number of other posts; Consulting Surgeon to the Metropolitan Ear Nose and Throat Hospital, London, and Consulting Surgeon to the Italian Hospital, London.

Unfortunately Hamilton Bailey's life was marred by tragedy. In 1943 his only son aged fifteen, was killed in an appalling railway accident. In 1948 Bailey suffered a very serious mental breakdown, and manic

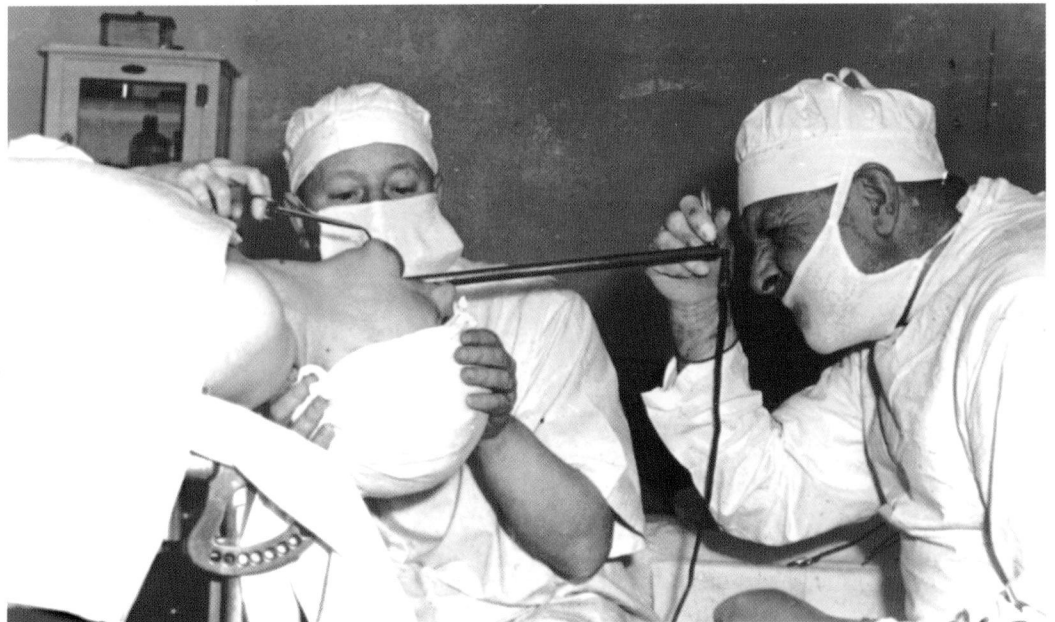

Hamilton Bailey using a rigid gastroscope Royal Northern Hospital, late 1930s.
Courtesy Royal London Hospital Archives ©

depression was diagnosed. He was admitted to a mental hospital and the prognosis was considered to be very poor, and in 1949 he resigned from the Royal Northern Hospital. During his last admission in 1951, at Graylingwell Mental Hospital, Chichester, a leucotomy was considered because of his deteriorating condition, but his wife Veta refused to consent to this procedure. In 1948 Dr John Cadet, working in an Australian psychiatric hospital, discovered and pioneered the use of Lithium salts (Lithium carbonate), in patients suffering from manic-depression. A very knowledgeable registrar at Graylingwell Hospital suggested the use of Lithium and it was decided to try this drug on Hamilton Bailey. This resulted in a considerable improvement in his mental state.

The Baileys retired to Spain in 1960 but in 1961 he developed symptoms of an intestinal obstruction due to a malignancy. Apparently Bailey interfered with the management of his case, which resulted in a number of unnecessary operations. Sadly he succumbed and died in Malaga, 26 March 1961.

Hamilton Bailey's fourteen books went through numerous editions, and were translated into many languages. Robert J McNeill Love was Bailey's principal co-author. Although Hamilton Bailey died more than forty years ago, new versions are still published under his name. The latest 24th edition of Bailey & Love's *Short Practice of Surgery* was published in 2004 and the tome has three editors and many contributors. The books remain popular in the developing world and the Hamilton Bailey Memorial Trust was established in 1967 to provide surgeons, teachers and students throughout the world, but particularly in third world countries, with surgical and medical textbooks and related media. The Trust is endowed partly through royalties on his publications.

Hamilton Bailey could well be regarded as one of the greatest surgical teachers of the 20th century.

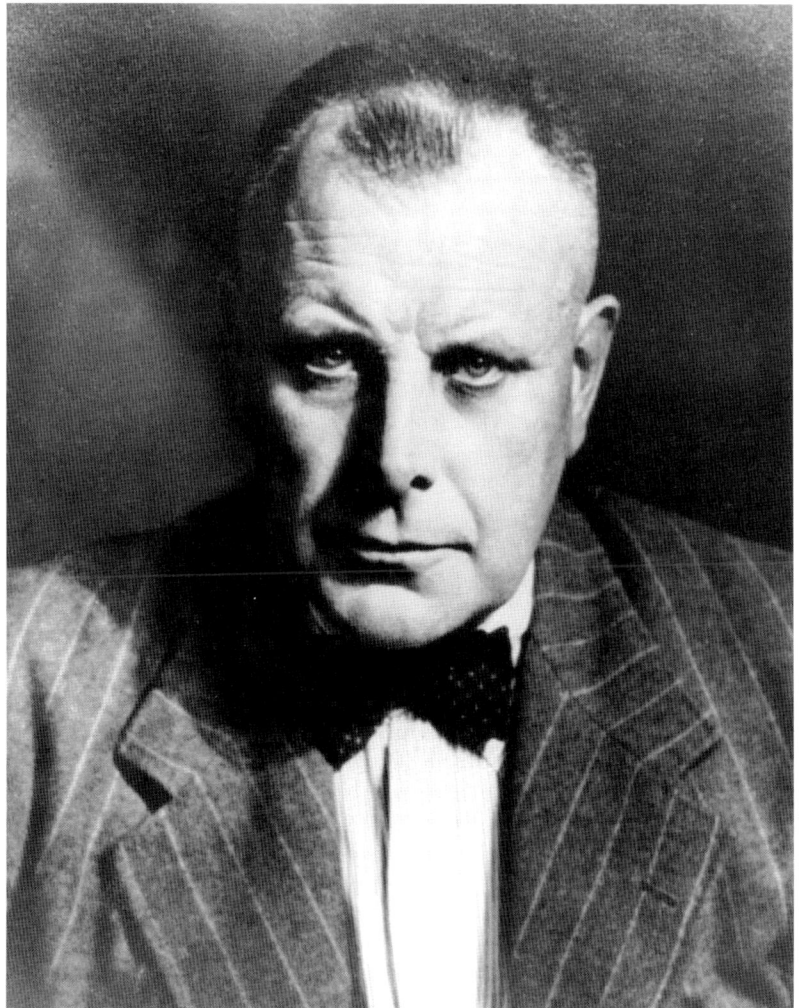

Hamilton Bailey FRCS, from an original portrait photograph which hung in the old Board Room of the Royal Northern Hospital.
Courtesy the Royal Northern Hospital Archives, Whittington Hospital

Robert John McNeill Love MS FRCS (1891–1974)

15

Robert John McNeill Love was born in Devonport on 2 May 1891. His father Joseph Boyd Love JP, was an Ulsterman who came to England penniless but eventually built up a highly successful firm in Plymouth. His mother Elizabeth Coleman, was a farmer's daughter. At one time the family lived at 'Outlands' a house in Devonport, formerly owned by 'Captain Scott of Antarctic' fame. The house was destroyed in World War II.

McNeill Love studied at the London Hospital graduating in 1914. He served in the RAMC throughout the First World War as a surgical specialist in India, the Dardanelles and the Middle East.

On demobilisation in 1919 he held junior surgical appointments at Poplar Hospital completing his final FRCS in 1920 and his London MS in 1921. He returned to the London Hospital and became chief assistant during the same period as Hamilton Bailey, but neither managed to obtain a consultant appointment. Was it serendipity, or astuteness on the part of the appointments committee, that in 1930 they were both appointed consultants at the Royal Northern Hospital? There was a long spell of successful collaboration that began by the publication of their *Short Practice of Surgery* in 1932, a book that reached its sixteenth edition in 1974. This book was translated into Italian, Spanish and Turkish. In 1933 Hamilton Bailey and McNeill Love published *Surgery for Nurses*, which ran into six editions.

McNeill Love served as Chairman of the Court of Examiners of the Royal College of Surgeons

Robert McNeill Love MS FRCS.
Reproduced by kind permission of the President &
Council of the Royal College of Surgeons of England

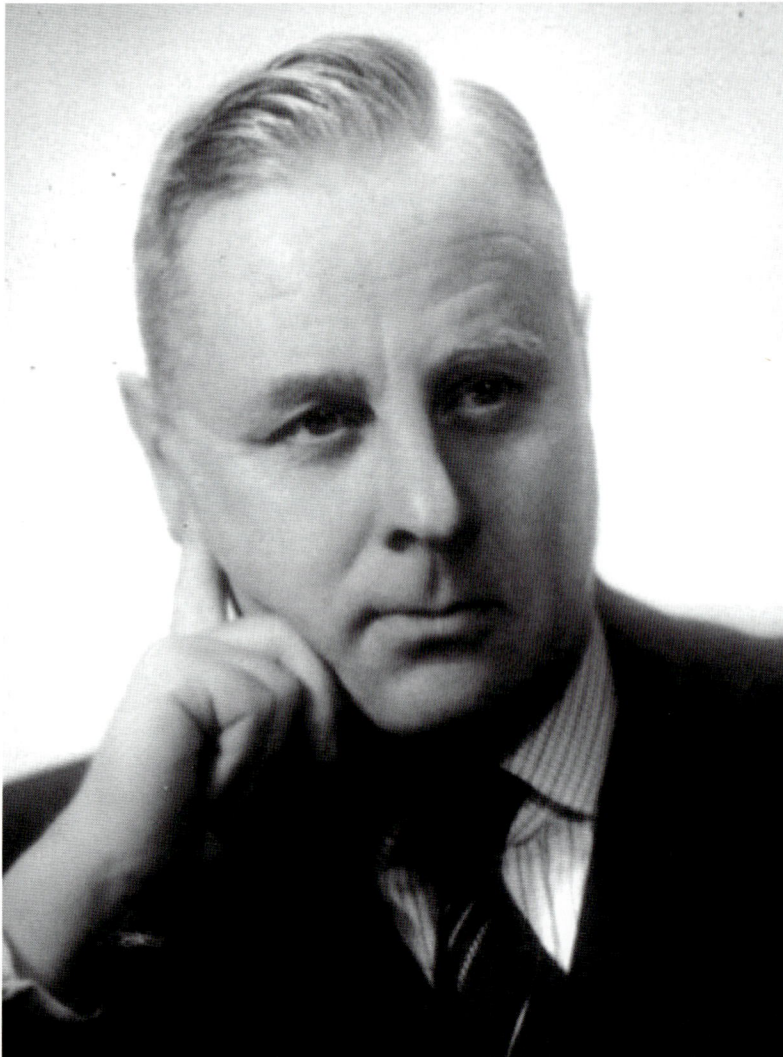

and was also a Member of Council from 1945–1953. He was a Hunterian Professor, and Erasmus Wilson Demonstrator.

'Robbie' as he was affectionately known, was a born teacher and an enthusiastic surgical tutor all his professional life. He was very much a general surgeon with a particular interest in the biliary tract and the thyroid gland. He was one of the first to use pre-operative cholangiography in England. He often said that, having been brought up in the days when it would be harmful to spend more than an hour in the abdomen, he found it hard to adjust to the slower and more precise operating conditions permitted by modern anaesthesia. He was also on the staff of the Metropolitan Hospital, the City of London Maternity Hospital and the West End Hospital for Nervous Diseases. After his retirement from the Royal Northern Hospital in 1956 and following the death of Hamilton Bailey, two reconstructed theatres were named after them.

Robert McNeill Love was married twice, first to Dorothy Borland in 1930 and after her death in 1961, he married Rhoda Mackie in the following year. His daughter by his first wife trained as a nurse and became head of the department of sociology at the North London Polytechnic, and in 1982 was created a Life Peer in the name of Baroness Cox.

Robert McNeill Love was a lover of country life and a staunch conservationist and an active Vice-President of the Hertfordshire Society. On retirement he farmed near Brickendon, Hertfordshire. Sadly he died on 1 October 1974 of an inoperable carcinoma of the stomach.

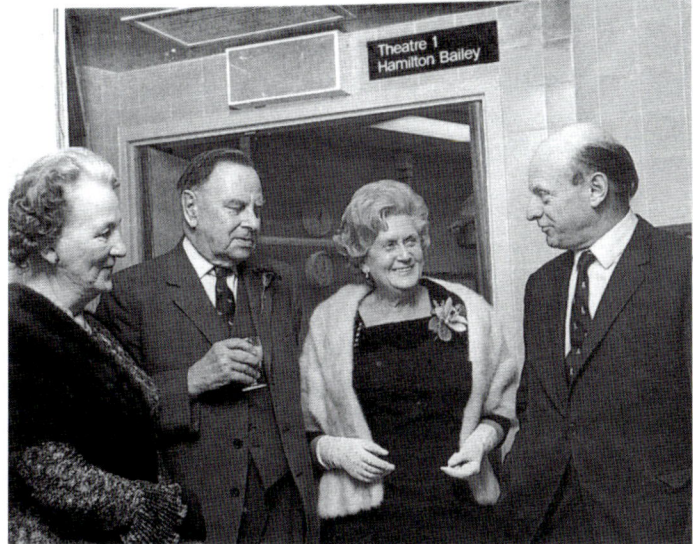

ISLINGTON GAZETTE TUESDAY OCTOBER 12 1971—FIVE

Hospital honours surgeons

Mrs Veta Hamilton Bailey stands beneath the nameplate of a theatre in the St. David's Wing of the Royal Northern Hospital, Holloway Road — the theatre named after her late husband, a surgeon. Mrs Hamilton Bailey was there to undertake, along with surgeon Mr Robbie McNeill Love, the opening of the Hamilton Bailey theatre and one named after Mr McNeill Love (second left). The two theatres have been upgraded at a cost of £85,000. Also in the picture for the re-opening of the upgraded theatres are Mrs Rhoda McNeill Love and consultant surgeon Mr Reg Murley.

Picture: Ray Lowe

Robert McNeill Love opening the refurbished operating theatre named after Hamilton Bailey, September 1971. From left to right: Rhoda and Robert McNeill Love, Veta Hamilton Bailey and Reginald Murley.
Courtesy Ray Lowe, Islington Gazette 1971

Sir Reginald Murley KBE TD MS FRCS (1916–1997)

16

Reginald Sidney Murley was born in Wandsworth on 2 August 1916. His father was a hide and skin warehouseman but rose to become the general manager of the Hudson Bay Company. His mother, Beatrice Bayliss, was a cousin of Lillian Bayliss, founder of The Old Vic.

One of Reginald Murley's earliest memories was having his tonsils removed on the kitchen table, during which he nearly asphyxiated! After leaving Dulwich College, he studied medicine at St Bartholomew's Hospital, gaining scholarships in anatomy and physiology in successive years. In May 1939 he graduated MB BS with honours in medicine and surgery. As a Territorial he joined the 168 City of London Cavalry Field Ambulance. Starting in a cavalry regiment he also learned to ride a horse, but his first experience was not a happy one as he was swept off his mount when it bolted and dragged him through a line of washing! During the Second World War he saw service in the Middle East, North Africa, Holland and Germany, and he gained valuable experience in the management of craniofacial injuries and orthopaedic trauma and in plastic surgery. Following demobilisation he gained a great deal of postgraduate training in general surgery. He passed the FRCS in 1946 and the MS (Master of Surgery) in 1948.

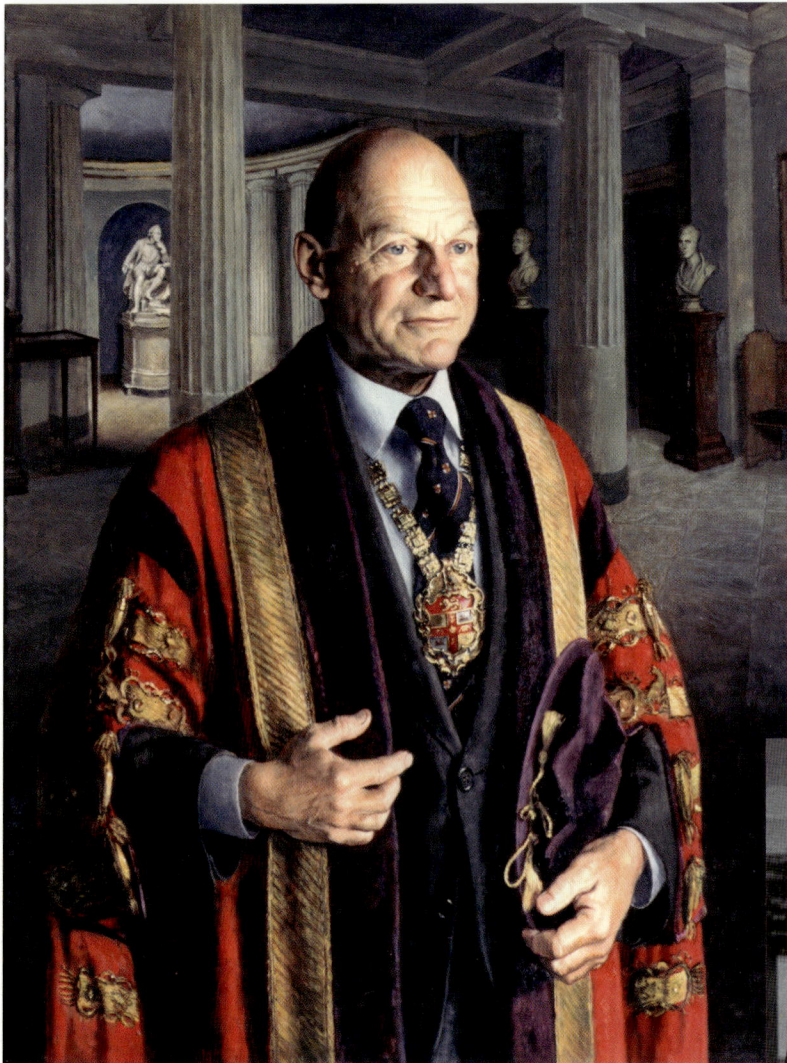

President of the Royal College of Surgeons of England, 1977-1980.
Portrait in oils 1982, John Walton RP

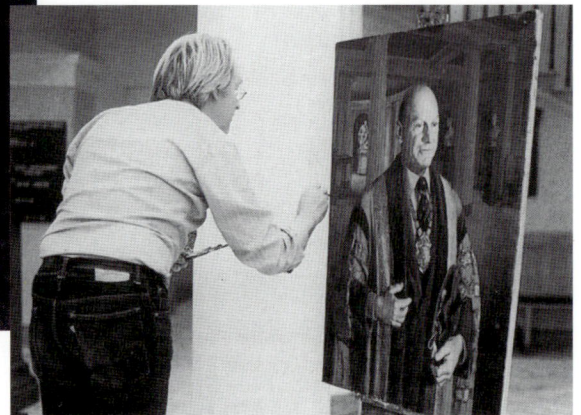

In 1947 he married Daphne Garrod who was then a young widow with a four-year-old daughter, both her previous husbands having been killed during the War.

In 1950 Reginald Murley became a Hunterian Professor at the Royal College of Surgeons. This was awarded for his excellent work on the detection and prevention of venous thrombosis. In 1953 he was appointed to the staff of St Albans Hospital and the Royal Northern Hospital, where he practised surgery to a very high standard. He loved teaching, but stated that he would not have been happy in a teaching hospital, much preferring to teach medical students and surgical trainees either individually or in very small groups.

Chairman of Trustees of the Hunterian Collection still displayed in the splendid refurbished Hunterian museum at the Royal College of Surgeons, London (*John Hunter was a leading London surgeon, anatomist, physiologist and pathologist of outstanding merit 1728-1793*).

In 1981 Sir Reginald Murley retired from the Royal Northern Hospital and in the following year he was elected President of the Medical Society of London.

In his last years, he was dogged by ill health, but in spite of this he took on many commitments including the chairmanship of the Medical Council on Alcoholism. Sir Reginald Murley died in 1997 at the age of eighty-one.

'He was a man of extraordinary vitality and energy outspoken and challenging, but with endless kindness, particularly to his juniors.'

The Times Obituary

Despite his involvement in medical politics he was always first and foremost a practising surgeon. In 1970 he was elected to the Council of the Royal College of Surgeons, and in 1977 he had the special honour of being elected President of the College and was knighted in 1979.

In the 1980s he gave some welcome publicity to the conservative local surgery for breast cancer in preference to radical mastectomy that was pioneered by Sir Geoffrey Keynes as far back as the 1920s. 'Reggie' Murley's great hero was John Hunter, and he became

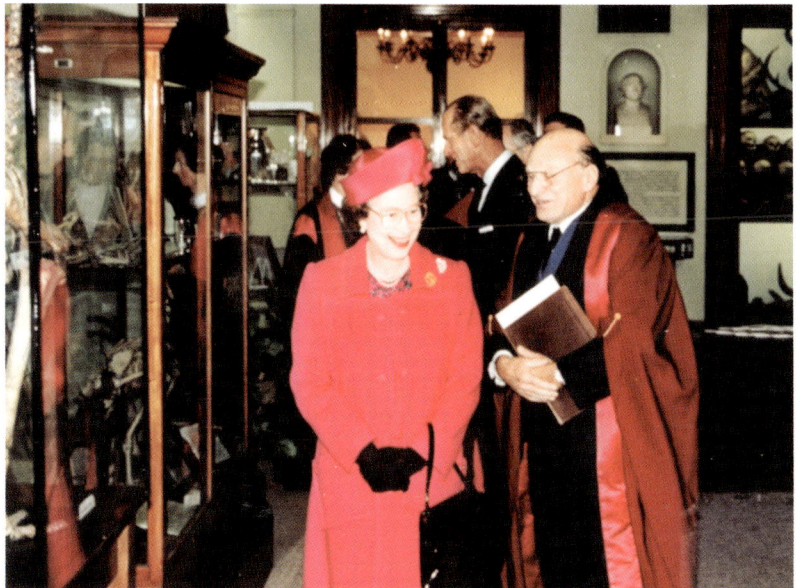

Visit to the Hunterian Museum, by HM Queen Elizabeth and Prince Philip with Sir Reginald Murley at the Royal College of Surgeons, 21 November 1989.

Images reproduced by kind permission of the President and Council of the Royal College of Surgeons of England

The Royal Northern Hospital – **World War II**

17 The Blitz was the sustained bombing of the United Kingdom by Nazi Germany between September 1940 and May 1941. Concentrated direct bombing of industrial targets and civilian centres began on 7 September 1940.

The scale of the attacks rapidly escalated, but the main attack was concentrated on London.

In September alone, the German Air Force dropped 5,300 tons of high explosives on London, in twenty-four nights. The Blitz inflicted around 43,000 deaths and destroyed over a million houses, but failed to achieve the Germans' strategic objectives of knocking Britain out of the war, or rendering it unable to resist an invasion.

Many organisations combined to help the hospitals through the difficult days of World War II. British and American Charities helped, including the American Red Cross Committee.

Money was sent, as well as surgical instruments which were most useful. Other American organisations which gave aid were 'Bundles for Britain Inc.', which sent clothing for patients, and the American War Relief Society who sent linen and other gifts.

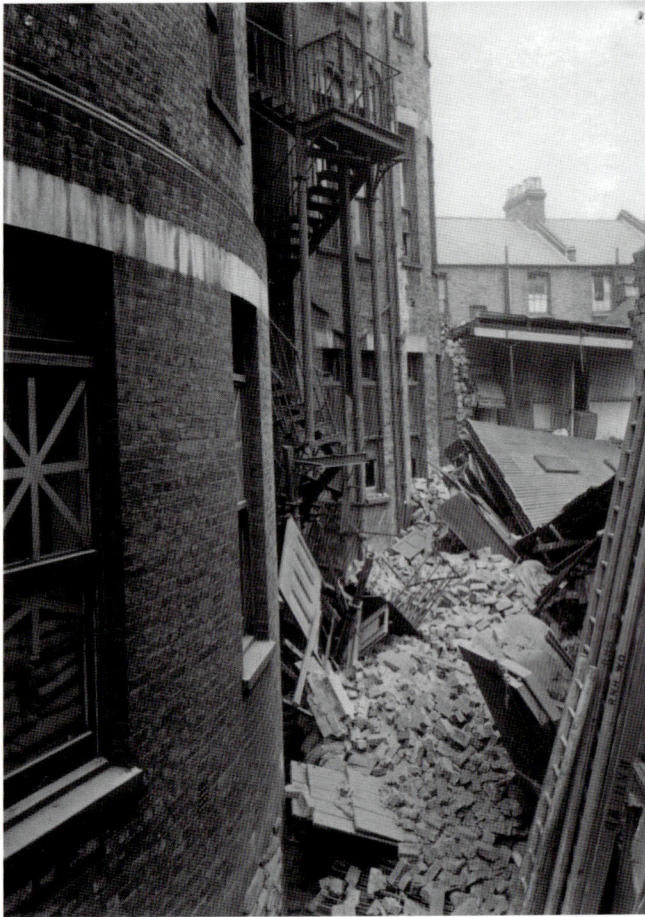

Part of the damage done at the hospital during an air raid in September 1940. The old boiler house and linen store were destroyed but there were no casualties.

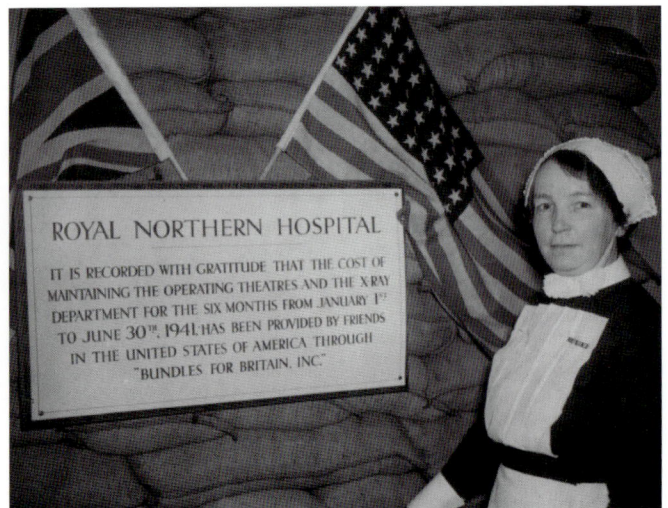

'Bundles for Britain Inc'.

An original enterprise which started in 1929, was the Royal Northern School of Housekeeping and Catering. Girls over sixteen years of age, who had obtained the school certificate, received a two years course, training in institutional management. This included catering, cooking, dietetics, home-nursing and general housekeeping duties. No fees were charged and the girls received free board, lodging and uniforms. Certificates were issued to all who had satisfactorily completed the course. The School flourished for the next 25 years until it gradually came to an end.

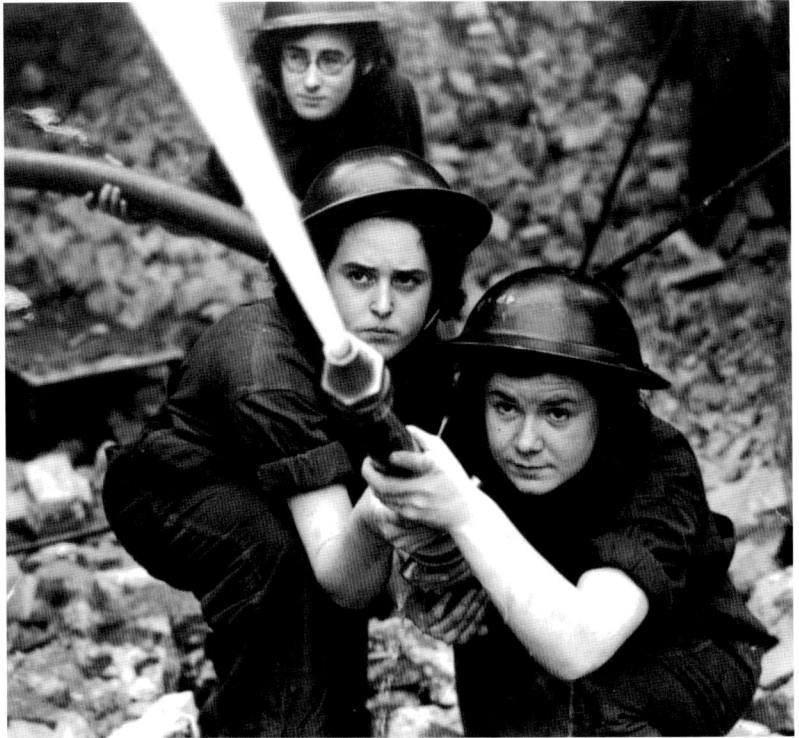

Fire-fighting teams at practice in World War II, made up by housekeeping students of the Royal Northern Hospital.

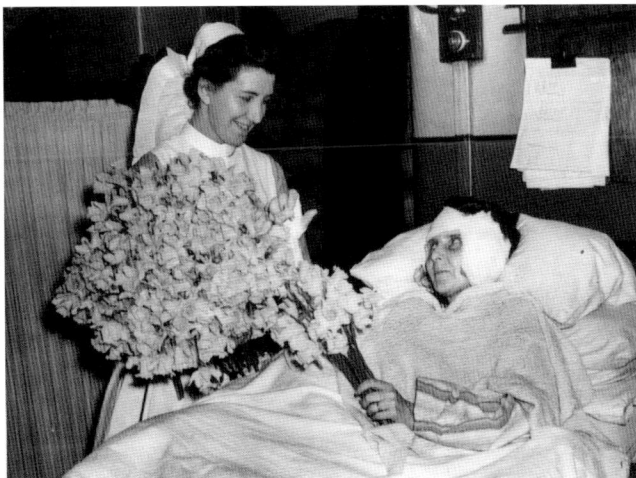

A patient injured in an air-raid, admiring spring flowers sent by their Majesties King George VI and Queen Elizabeth.
Courtesy Fox Photos Ltd

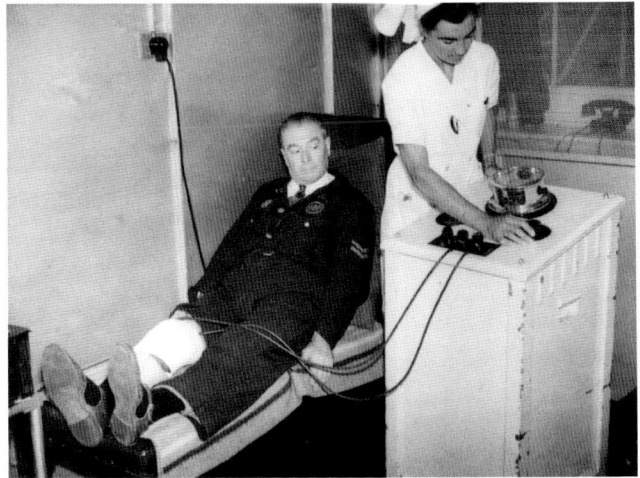

1940s, Physiotherapist treats the patient with faradism, (the use of pulsed or AC current to stimulate muscle contraction). The patient was in the Air Raid Precautions (ARP) organisation.
Courtesy Fox Photos Ltd

Photographs courtesy the Royal Northern Hospital Archives, Whittington Hospital

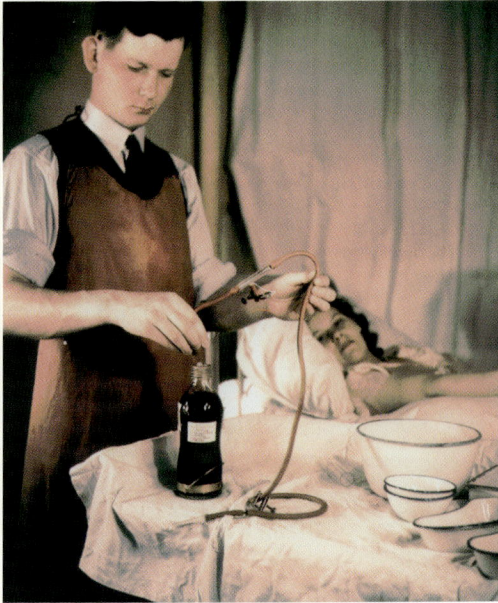

Doctor attaches transfusion apparatus to blood bottle.

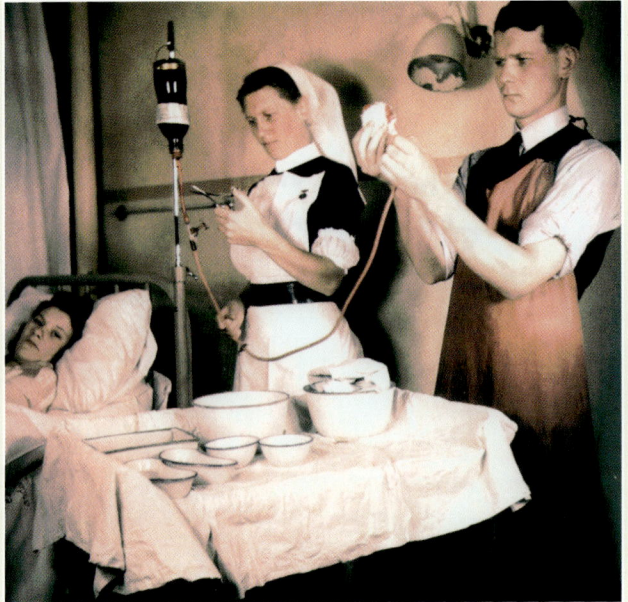

Blood transfusion procedure.

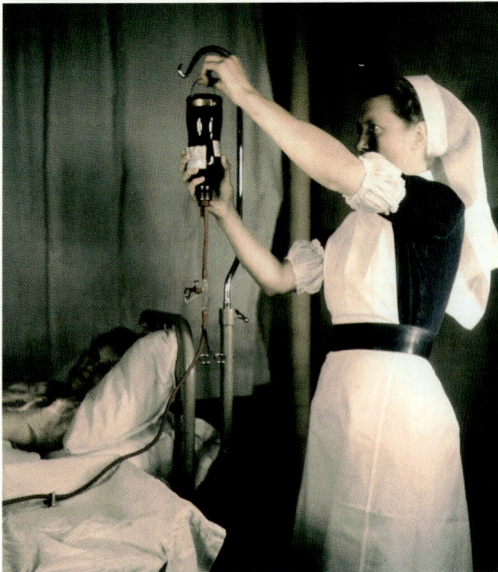

Sister adjusts blood bottle for transfusion.

Royal Northern Hospital c.1940s
Hamilton Bailey Collection.
©The Royal London Hospital Archives

The Royal Chest Hospital, City Road

18

The Royal Chest Hospital was founded in 1814 by Dr Isaac Buxton (1775–1825). He started life as a non-conformist minister but subsequently turned to medicine and in 1802, graduated MD Göttingen, Germany. In 1807 he was appointed physician to the London Hospital but resigned in 1822 because of strained relations with the governors. Dr Isaac Buxton was struck by the fact that there were separate hospitals for many diseases and although there was a high death rate from pulmonary diseases there was no institution where the treatment for pulmonary disease 'could have a fair and persevering trial'. He advocated a moderate summer temperature of 60–65°F in the wards all the year round, combined with skilled nursing, and he founded the hospital principally for that reason. It is generally regarded that this was the first chest hospital in the world. Its original name was the Infirmary for Asthma, Consumption and other Pulmonary Diseases. Later the 'Heart and Great Vessels' was incorporated into the name and in 1848 Queen Victoria bestowed the Royal title to the chest hospital.

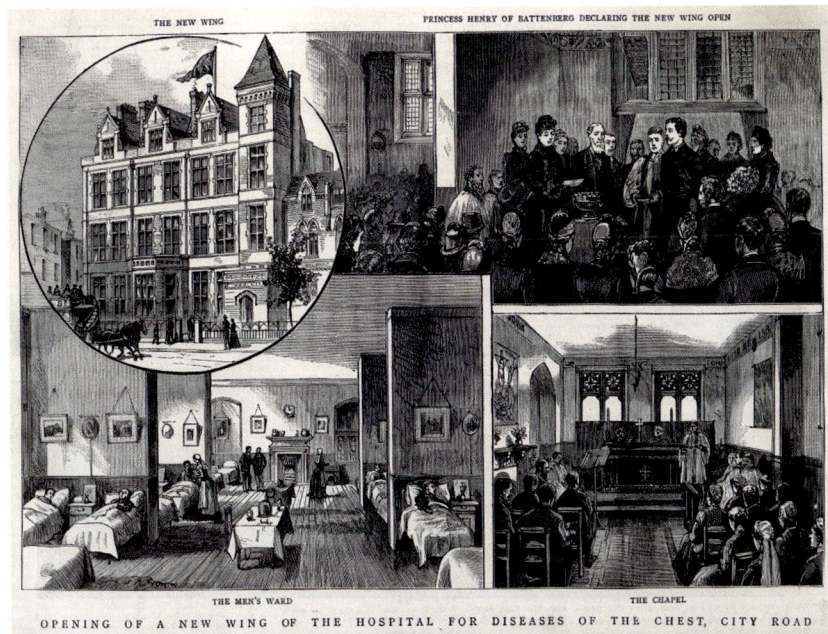

THE NEW WING

PRINCESS HENRY OF BATTENBERG DECLARING THE NEW WING OPEN

THE MEN'S WARD

THE CHAPEL

OPENING OF A NEW WING OF THE HOSPITAL FOR DISEASES OF THE CHEST, CITY ROAD

The new wing was opened by Prince Henry of Battenberg (c.1885) who was married to Princess Beatrice, youngest daughter of Queen Victoria.

Courtesy the Wellcome Library

The hospital began in a twelve-room house in Union Street (now Brushfield Street), Bishopsgate and after several moves, finally in 1849, settled in City Road in a house belonging to St Bartholomew's Hospital. The chest hospital bought the leasehold in 1880.

In 1862 the house in City Road was pulled down and a building more suitable for a hospital was erected, and in 1880 further extensions were made completing the familiar frontal appearance.

In 1912 the tuberculosis dispensary for the boroughs of Islington, Shoreditch and Finsbury was housed in the hospital. In 1919 it became known as the Royal Chest Hospital but, because of financial difficulties, the hospital amalgamated with the Great Northern Hospital which acquired a title and paid its debts. The medical staff at the Royal Chest Hospital continued their work independently and unimpaired until the Second World War.

Air-Raid 1940

On 11 September 1940 the hospital had a direct hit. A bomb crashed through the front of the hospital, shattering all the wards. Under the most terrible conditions, the whole staff, all of whom were injured, worked quickly and calmly in rescuing patients, who

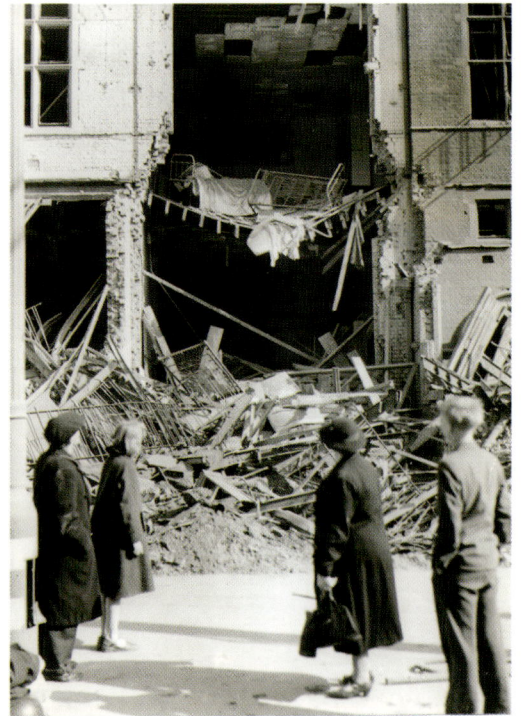

A first floor ward of the in-patients department of the Hospital, exposed to view of pedestrians in the City Road, after a direct hit by a bomb on the night of 11 September 1940.

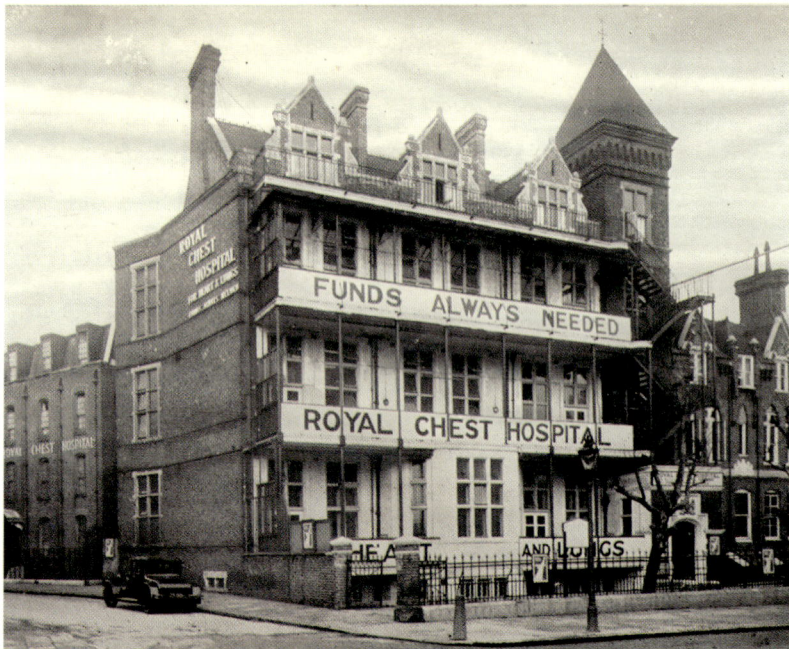

Royal Chest Hospital, Annual Report 1932.

Images courtesy the Royal Northern Hospital Archives, Whittington Hospital

were also injured. The resident engineer Mr A E Davis of the Royal Chest Hospital was killed. Only a few nights previously he had led others in saving the hospital, which had been hit with incendiary bombs.

The hospital staff were joined by doctors and nurses from the Royal Northern Hospital to help in the rescue of the injured among the debris. All the staff showed outstanding courage and devotion to duty; no patient's life was lost. HM King George VI awarded the George Medal to three members of staff of the Royal Chest Hospital for their outstanding bravery; the recipients were Dr Andre Bathfield (Resident Medical Officer), Miss Catherine McGovern (Acting Matron) and Nurse Patricia Marmion.

The out-patients department continued to function until the hospital was finally demolished in 1954. The hospital was never rebuilt.

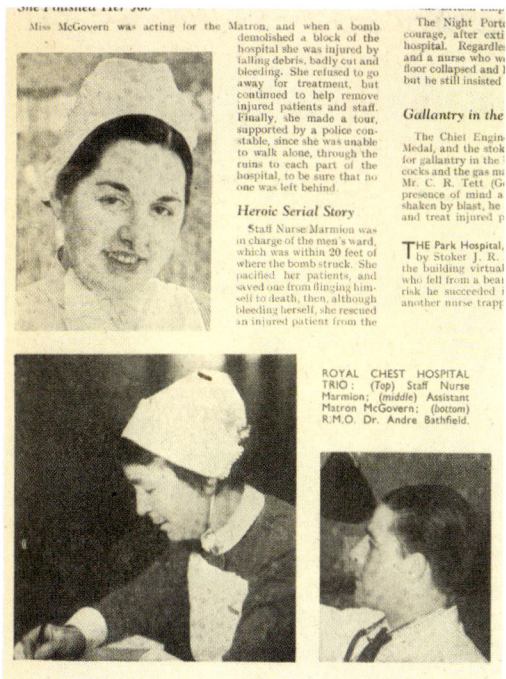

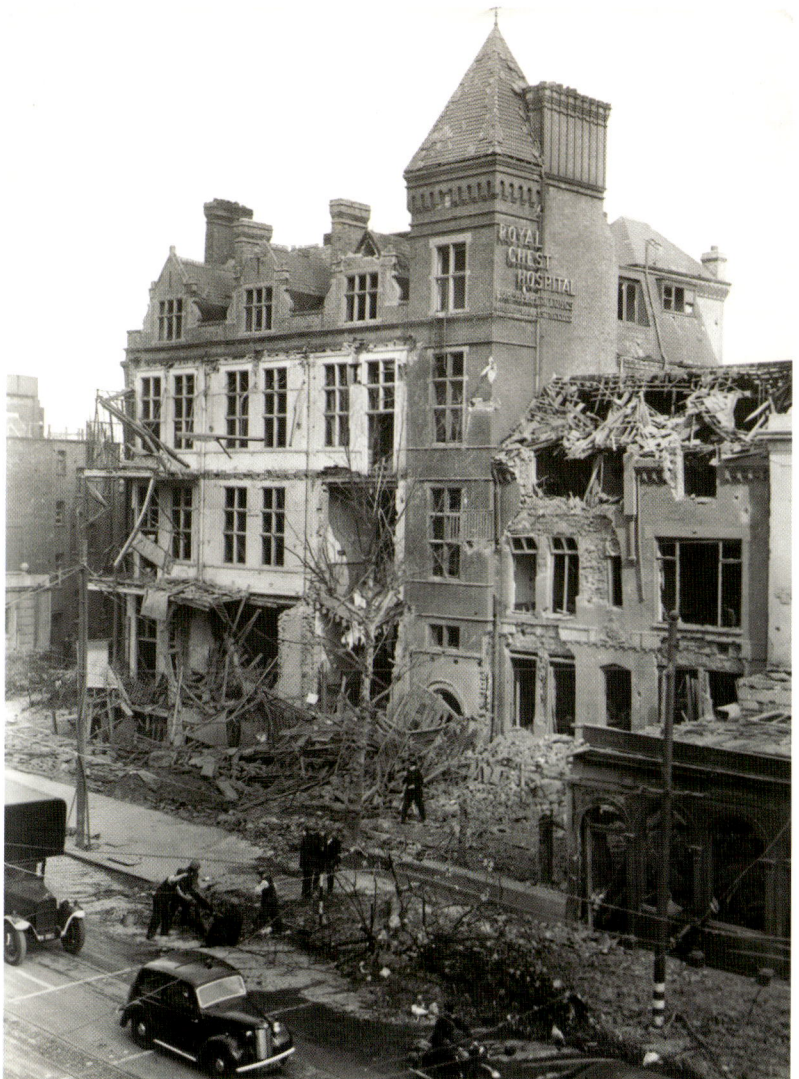

Staff Nurse Marmion (top), Assistant Matron McGovern (bottom left), Dr Andre Bathfield (bottom right). The Nursing Mirror 25 January 1941.
By permission of the British Library.
Picture no 1007628.021 BL. Ref. NPL

The bombed Royal Chest Hospital, City Road, September 1940.
Courtesy Royal Northern Hospital Archives, Whittington Hospital

City of London Maternity Hospital 1750–1983

19

The City of London Maternity Hospital was founded in 1750 as a… 'Lying-in Hospital for Married Women in the City of London, and parts adjacent, and also for Sick and Lame Out-Patients… an apartment to be taken in London House, Aldersgate Street, to be converted into proper wards for this Lying-In Hospital…' The next year in 1751, the hospital moved to Shaftesbury House, still in Aldersgate Street, and changed its name to the 'City of London Lying-in-Hospital for Married Women.' In 1770 the hospital moved to a new site on the corner of City Road and Old Street.

Dr John Coakley Lettsom (1744–1815), the distinguished eighteenth century Quaker doctor was physician to the City of London Lying-in Hospital from 1785–1815. He was the founder of the Medical Society of London.

In 1907 the greater part of the old hospital was pulled down, and rebuilt on the same site in City Road. In 1918, at the suggestion of the Ladies Association, it was decided to change the name of the hospital to the City of London Maternity Hospital, on the grounds that the words 'Lying-in' were unpleasant to the modern ear.

Some institutions outlive their usefulness, or the purpose for which they were formed fails. It may, with perfect truth, however be claimed for the City of London Maternity Hospital, that, needed as it possibly was in 1750, it was never more needed than at the present day. The surrounding neighbourhoods of Finsbury, Islington, Bethnal Green and Shoreditch are of the poorest, and it is from these that the bulk of its patients are drawn. Whatever the future may have in store for the Voluntary Hospitals, there remains the fact that a considerable proportion of the patients who apply to this institution for relief, live from hand to mouth with little or no margin of income above the poverty line. For such was this Hospital founded, and for such it exists today, a haven of rest for the toiling mother at the critical period of childbirth, or on whose behalf are enlisted the resources of Medical and Nursing Science.

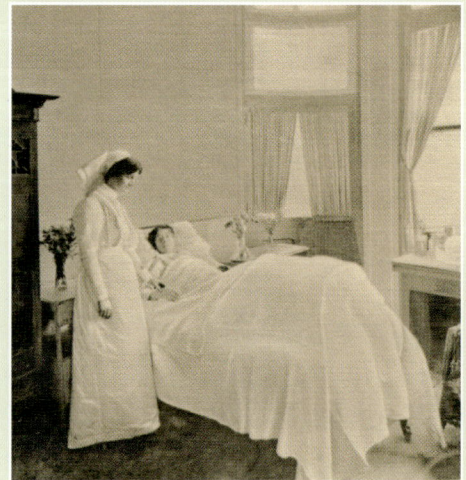

A private room

Extract from 'The City of London Maternity Hospital A Short History' *by Ralph B Cannings 1922, Secretary to the Hospital (1919–1944). Published privately*

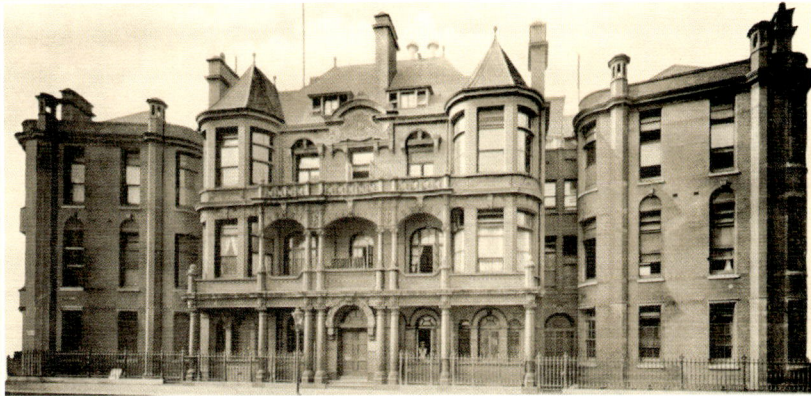

The front of the Hospital

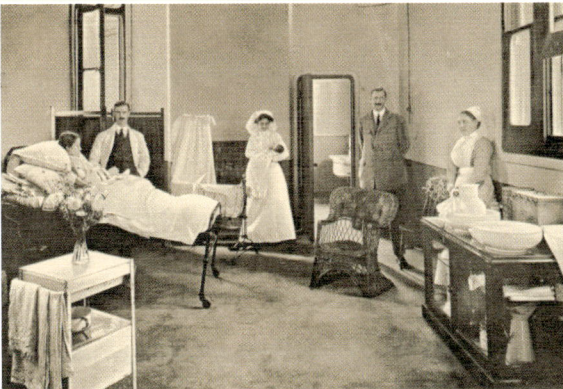

Isolation ward

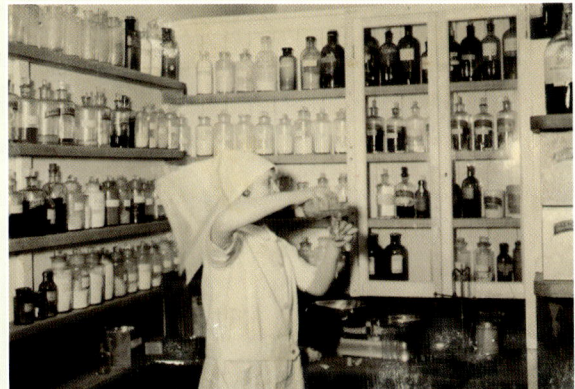

The pharmacy

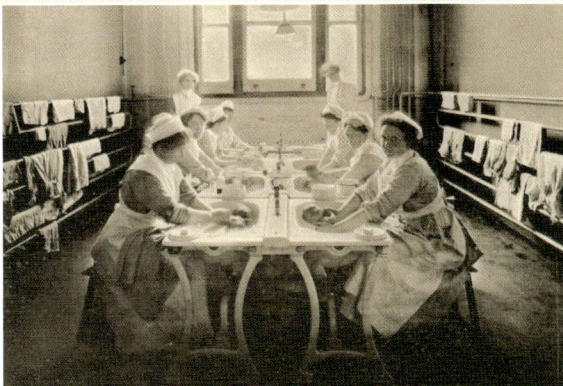

A babies' bath room

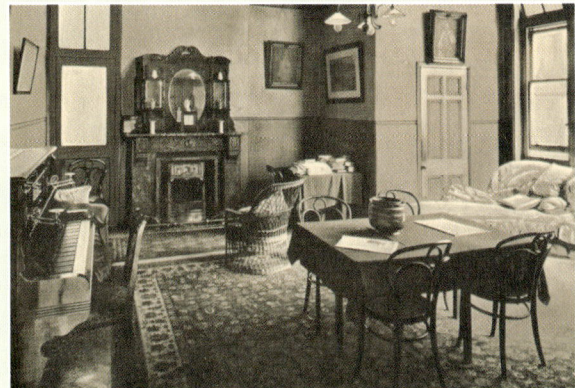

Nurses' sitting room

Photographs early 1900s, courtesy Royal Northern Hospital Archives, Whittington Hospital

The hospital in the 'Blitz'

It was the evening of 9 September 1940 and in accordance with nightly ritual, mothers and babies had been brought downstairs to the ground floor of the hospital main corridor, and made comfortable on mattresses. The 'red' warning came through and shortly afterwards hell seemed to be let loose over London. Suddenly there was a sickening crash overhead. A high explosive bomb fell and struck the northern wing of the hospital building, demolishing it from roof to basement.

Immediately the lights in the corridor went out and the air was filled with choking dust from the falling masonry and ceilings, but there was no panic The devastation was only about a dozen yards from where the mothers were lying, but the nursing staff moved calmly among the mothers and babies, (with the aid of torches) ministering to their comfort. Evacuation was arranged quickly, and with the arrival of ambulances, the transfer temporarily to Friern Barnet Hospital, in North London, was effected amid continuous gunfire overhead. The only casualty was a nurse with a slightly injured arm. The demolished wing included two eight-bed wards and some single bedrooms beneath. The blast had made a shambles of two labour wards and admission of patients to the hospital had become impracticable Those applying were accordingly evacuated to Brocket Hall, Hertfordshire or sent to the hospital's temporary accommodation at Friern Hospital.

In anticipation of the outbreak of war, Brocket Hall a stately mansion near Welwyn Garden City, had been taken over by the Board of Management and equipped; it became fully operational on the outbreak of war.

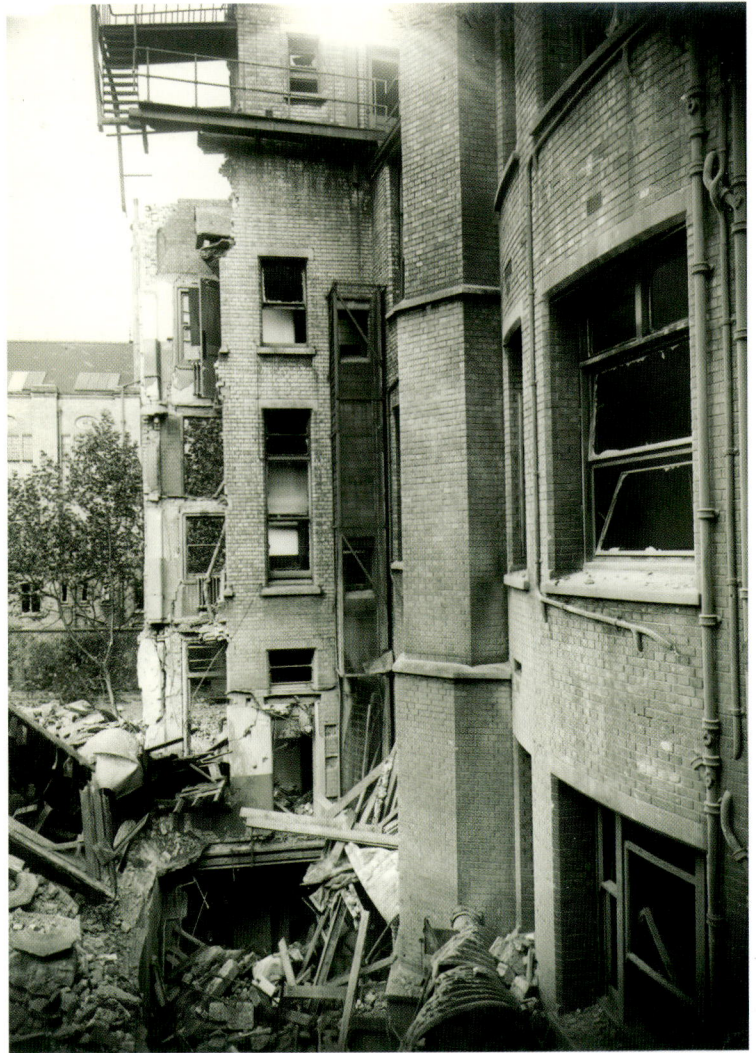

Where the bomb fell 9 September 1940, demolishing the Northern Wing.
Courtesy Photopress Ltd and the Royal Northern Hospital Archives, Whittington Hospital

Extract from 'The City of London Maternity Hospital in the Blitz'*, by Ralph B. Cannings, Secretary to the Hospital. The Medical Press and Circular, June 1943*

The Amalgamation with the Royal Northern Hospital

'…*For a long time, the patients were accommodated at Brocket Hall, near Welwyn Garden City, Hertfordshire. In 1949 the North London Home for the Blind in Hanley Road, Upper Islington, was converted into accommodation for 52 in-patients. The altered building became the new home for the City of London Maternity Hospital near its new parent hospital, the Royal Northern Hospital. The official opening on 31 March 1950 coincided with the bi-centenary of the City of London Maternity Hospital, which finally closed its doors in 1983…*'

Extract from an unpublished account by Beryl Warner,
Secretary to the City of London Maternity Hospital 1963–1983

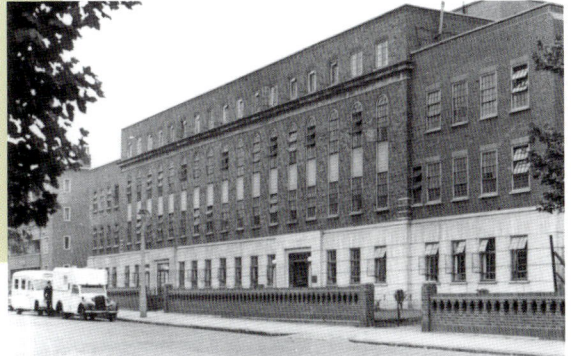

The City of London Maternity Hospital,
Hanley Road – 1950s

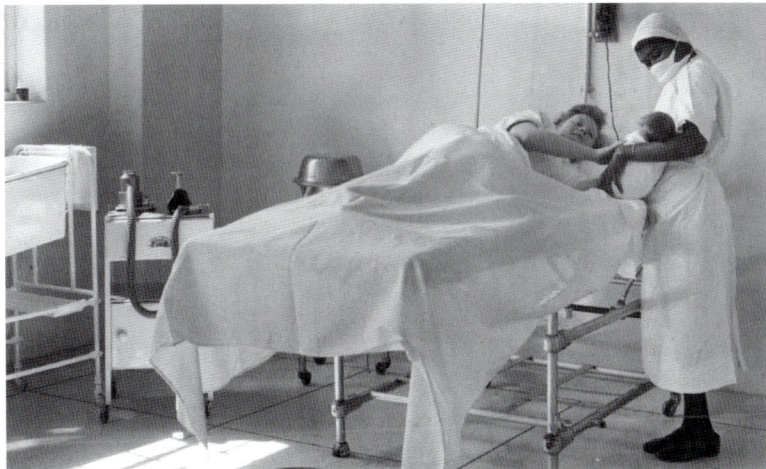

Delivery room, the City of London Maternity Hospital, Hanley Road,
Islington 1955. Courtesy Nucleus photographic Specialist Ltd.

The maternity unit of the Whittington Hospital was named the City of London Maternity Unit.

The traditions of the former City of London Maternity Hospital continue to thrive with the carc and modern technology at the Whittington Hospital, serving the large population of Islington and beyond.

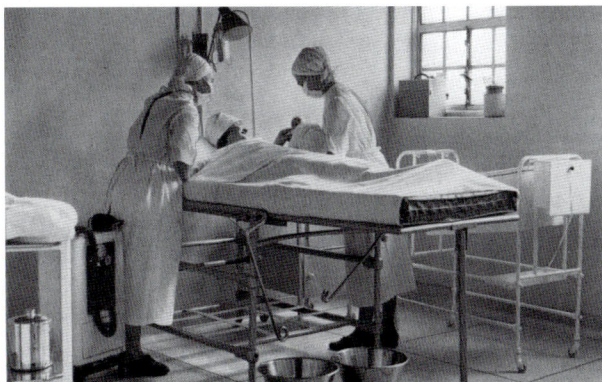

Mother's first introduction to her New Baby

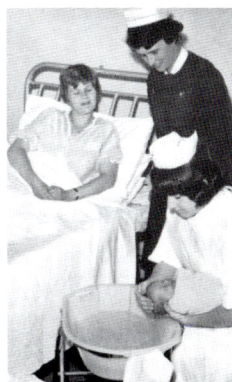

Mother's first lesson

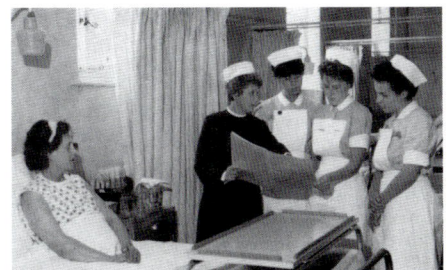

A bedside tutorial

Images Courtesy the Royal Northern Hospital Archives, Whittington Hospital

The Radiotherapy Department

20

Director: Dr Anthony Green FRCS FFR (died 3 September 1993)
Head of Medical Physics: Dr W Alan Jennings PhD FInstP FIPEM

In 1946 at the Royal Northern Hospital a Joint Radiotherapy Centre was formed, run in conjunction with the Prince of Wales General Hospital, Tottenham. By pooling the resources of the two hospitals in this way, access to a much larger range of expensive equipment became possible for the benefit of the patients in North London. The staff was enlarged to include full time physicists and the Centre made notable contributions to progress in radiotherapy. It was the first to have all types of moving-beam therapy in action. Much of the apparatus was designed at the Royal Northern Hospital and was adopted elsewhere. Advances were also made in the use of low-voltage radiation, radium, and radon seeds.

This department achieved an international reputation as a centre of innovation.

Many projects were presented and exhibited at a series of International Congresses of Radiology (1950-1959) and described in numerous publications.

Personal account by Dr Alan Jennings

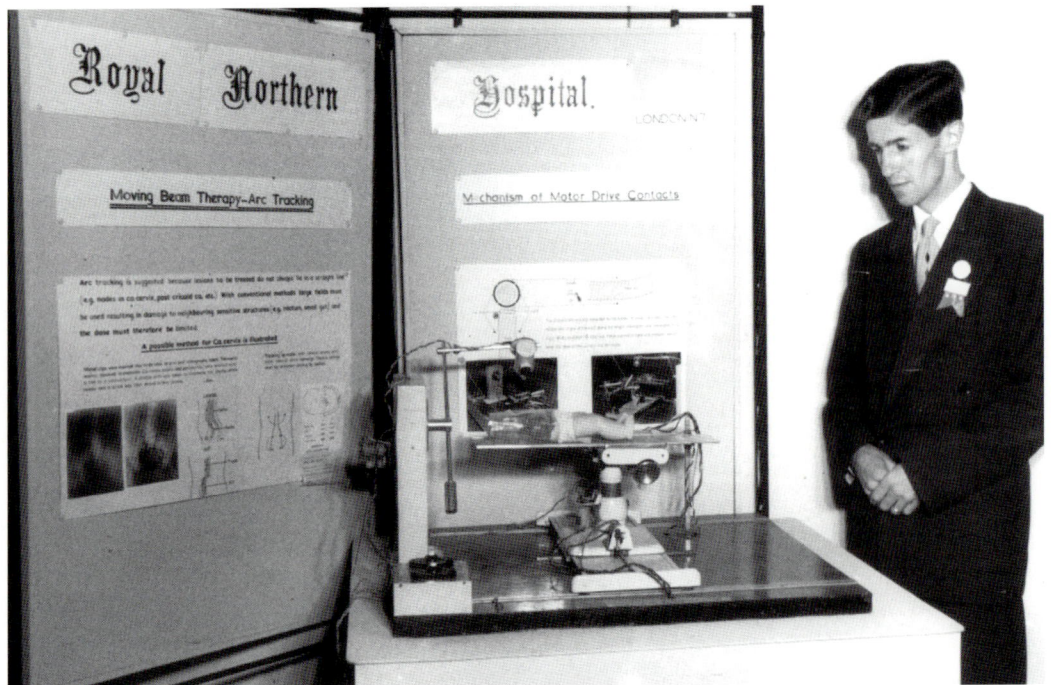

Dr W Alan Jennings with his exhibit; a model of equipment for 3D 'tracking irradiation'. The patient lies on a couch, which travels along rails under an 'arcing' beam. The couch moves sideways and vertically, to keep in focus along the line of tumour spread.

The Radiotherapy Department, Royal Northern Hospital at the International Congress of Radiology, Munich, 1959.

Photograph courtesy Dr W Alan Jennings PhD FInstP FIPEM

Kathleen Clara Clark MBE FSR FRPS (1896–1968)

21

The School of Radiography

Kathleen Clark was born at Fulham in 1898. She began her radiographic career at the age of twenty-three and began her training course at Guys Hospital. She passed the first qualifying examination ever held by the Society of Radiographers in 1922. Initially she worked at the Princess Mary's Hospital for Surgical Tuberculosis, and Margate General Hospital from 1922–1927.

She joined the Royal Northern Hospital in 1927 as a radiographer and was Radiographer-in-charge from 1927 to 1935. She was aware of the lack of adequate training for radiographers and founded a school of radiography in 1929. She was a gifted teacher and was tutor from 1930–1935. The School of Radiography at the Royal Northern Hospital was one of the earliest to be established in the country; the first was at the Royal Victoria Military Hospital, Netley, Southampton.

In 1935 she left to join Ilford Limited and became co-founder and Principal of the Ilford Radiographic Department which developed a worldwide reputation. She was involved in instruction in radiography and medical photography. 'Kitty' Clark became President of the Society of Radiographers 1935–1937 (also the first woman President). In 1939 her classic book, *Positioning in Radiography* was published which became the standard work of reference for radiographers and achieved universal acclaim. The artist Francis Bacon (1909–1992), acknowledged that her text-book, *Positioning in Radiography,* was a crucial source for his paintings. Lawrence Gowing* has indicated that Bacon repeatedly borrowed from the photographs in her book for his work.

Contribution by
Dr Adrian Thomas FRCP FRCR

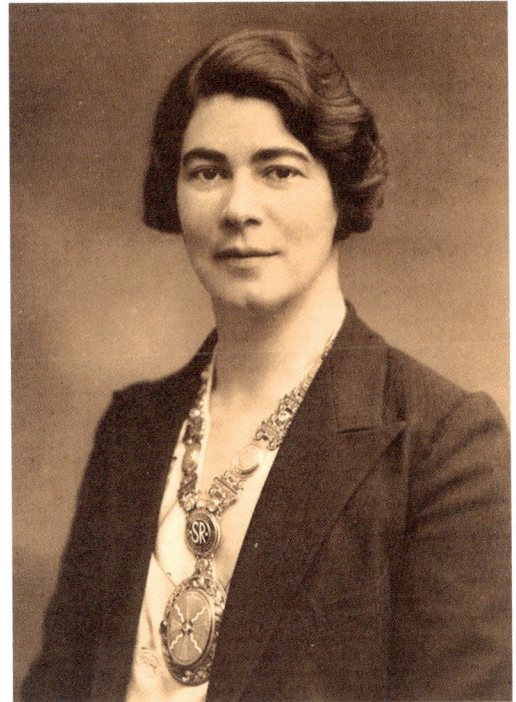

Kathleen Clark MBE FRPS FSR, President of the Society of Radiographers (1935–37).
Photograph courtesy the British Institute of Radiology

*Professor Sir Lawrence Gowing CBE RA (1918–1991). Slade Professor of Fine Art, University College London, 1975–85

During World War II Kathleen Clark worked in co-operation with the army medical services to perfect radiographic techniques for use in casualty clearing stations and she is associated, in a leading capacity, with the development of mass miniature radiography. By 1943, seventy mass miniature radiography units had been established throughout the country. She was awarded the MBE in 1945 for her services to radiography; particularly for mass miniature radiography of the chest. She played a vital role in the foundation of the International Society of Radiographers and Radiological Technologists (ISRRT), which was formally founded in 1962. Kathleen Clark died on 20 October 1968.

Kathleen Clark's obituary
Radiography Vol. XXXIV No.40 8 December 1968

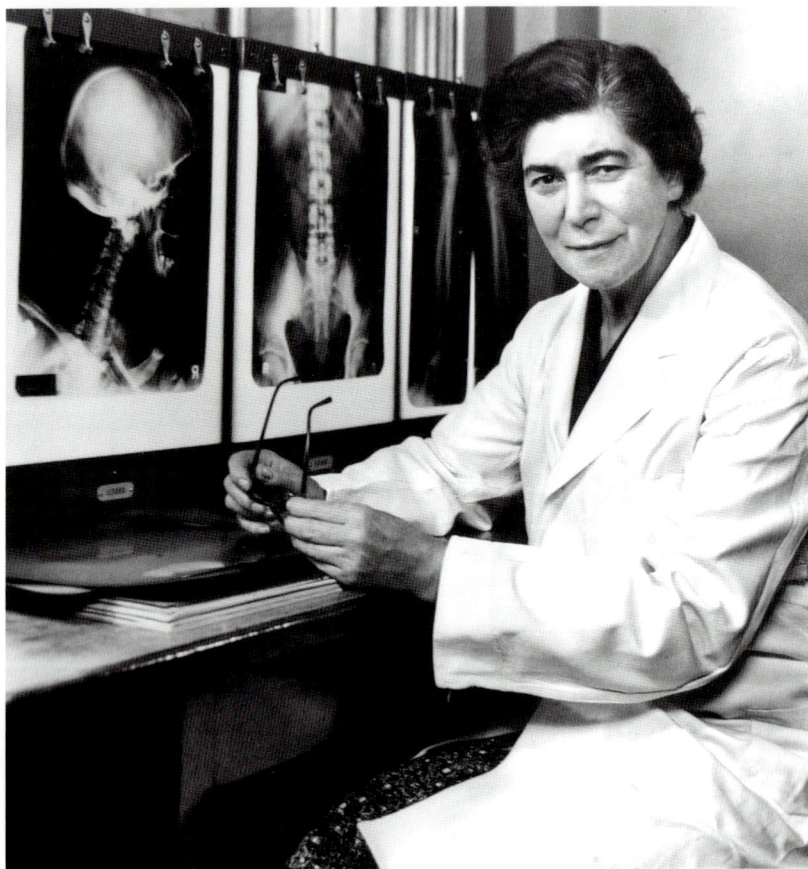

Kathleen Clark. c1950. Photo courtesy the British Institute of Radiology

'My memories of Miss K C Clark'
Marion Frank OBE Hon DSc Hon MSc FCR

In 1938, I came with my twin sister to England, as refugees from Nazi oppression. We were just eighteen. It was always our ambition to study medicine but because of financial reasons this was not possible. In 1938 we were living close to the Royal Northern Hospital and we were accepted as 'helpers' in the post-mortem room. We were introduced to Kathleen Clark who, although she had moved to the Ilford Radiographic Department, still retained connections with the Royal Northern Hospital. She suggested to us radiography as a profession. At that time the fee for training was £50 per annum and the period of training should have been eighteen months. However we had to interrupt our training as those of German origin were not allowed to study in central London, which was a prohibited area after May 1940. We joined our parents, who were now in Huddersfield, and applied to other training schools.

My sister and I completed our final six months at the Glasgow Western Infirmary, both passing the MSR in November 1941. I worked in Canada from 1948 to 1949, greatly encouraged in all my activities by Kathleen Clark, she being head of Ilford Ltd Education Department at Tavistock House. I became Superintendent and Principal of the School of Radiography at the Middlesex Hospital from 1949 until my retirement in 1981.

During the period at the Middlesex Hospital I had many contacts with Kathleen Clark as Tavistock House was close to The Middlesex Hospital and she on many occasions wanted to see specific procedures being performed.

Kathleen Clark was a founder member of the International Society of Radiographers and Radiological Technologists (ISRRT) in 1962 and was very influential in formulating the policies of the ISRRT, especially in the educational field. She appointed me to the Educational Committee and I became her successor as Chairman of the ISRRT Education Committee after her death in 1968.

As member of the Council and Education Committee of the Society of Radiographers I was their representative on the Royal Northern Hospital Radiographic Education Committee until 1980 under the Chairmanship of Dr Steve Carstairs (consultant radiologist).

Kathleen Clark's international connections were partly passed on to me and her personal interactions with colleagues in Australia and New Zealand continue to this day.

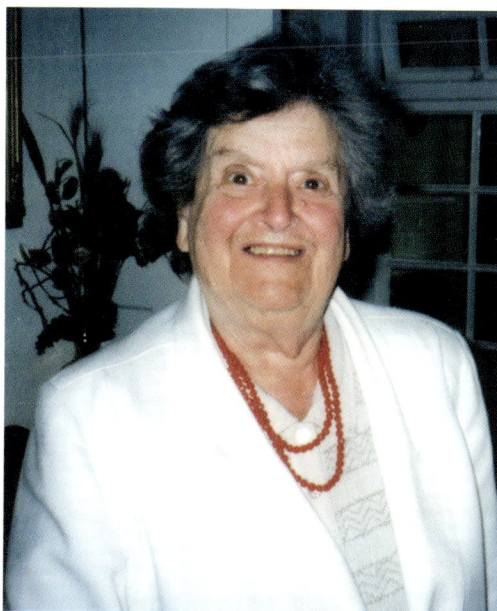

Marion Frank OBE FCR.
Photograph courtesy
Marion Frank 2006

Personal accounts of former consultants

22

The Department of Postgraduate Medical Education
Dr D Geraint James MD FRCP, Dean (1962–1985)

Throughout its life, the Royal Northern Hospital (Holloway Road) was a teaching hospital for medical students, postgraduate doctors, nurses, physiotherapists and for its own internal medical staff. This open house and free-for-all policy was understandable under the prevailing circumstances. In London, teaching hospitals were maintained for undergraduates and Hammersmith Hospital's Postgraduate Medical School was strictly for postgraduates. Where then did overseas students tend to congregate for further training? The Royal Northern Hospital certainly provided a ready clinical excellence and a wide-ranging programme of medical education.

Professor Om Sharma has described it as 'an inbuilt medical United Nations with a large flow of international visitors'. He described the weekly staff conferences

as occasions of sophisticated, intellectual debate lightened by agreeable repartee… the most lively and rewarding in Britain. During his three-year stay he met and exchanged ideas with Nobel Laureates, Peter Medawar (immunology), Baruch Blumberg (studies on hepatitis B), and geneticist Alexander Barn. He also met hepatologist Sheila Sherlock, gastro-enterologist Christopher Booth, and surgeon Arthur Dickson-Wright. Another eminent doctor he met was the distinguished cardiologist Sir John McMichael.

Postgraduate doctors needed the MRCP or the FRCS without delay and there was a high success rate for these and other diplomas. The surgeons Mr Hamilton Bailey and Mr McNeill Love were followed by the sharp wit and superb teaching of surgeon Mr Reginald Murley, later to become the President of The Royal College of Surgeons and to be honoured with a knighthood. Postgraduate doctors were from the old British Commonwealth, Australia, Africa, Hong Kong, Singapore, the Caribbean, as well as from the USA; they hastened home with their new degrees and set up consultant practices and new medical schools around the world.

Undergraduates needed an MB qualification, so the students attended ward rounds and out-patient clinics for extra tuition. When I was a medical student at the Middlesex Hospital I took advantage of the Royal Northern open house for further experience. Many found their way from the Royal Free Hospital and University College Hospital. It is probable that some would never have qualified but for this extra personalised tuition!

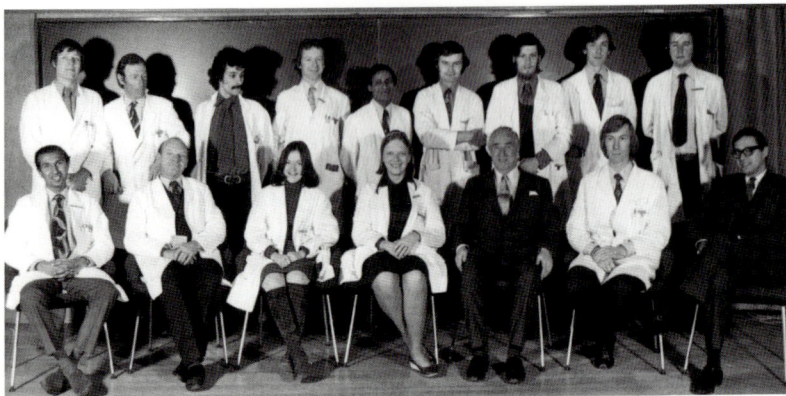

Group photo of postgraduate doctors and staff c1972. Dean, Dr Geraint James MD FRCP seated third from right; Mr Reginald Murley MS FRCS, senior surgeon, seated second from left; seated extreme right, Mr Trevor Dutt FRCOG then obstetric registrar.
Photo, courtesy Dr Geraint James MD FRCP

Dr Steve Carstairs provided a superb department of radiology. The same may be said for orthopaedic surgery, neurosurgery, obstetrics, gynaecology and paediatrics departments of medicine, surgery, anaesthetics, physiotherapy, dentistry and all other specialities provided a splendid service. What a pity it had to end!

Mr Ronald Miller MS FRCS FRGS. Urological Surgeon and Dean (1986–1992)

In 1986, I was appointed consultant urological surgeon to the Royal Northern Hospital to replace Mr Shuttleworth FRCS who had retired. Initially this was a shared appointment between the Institute of Urology, London and the Royal Northern Hospital. My appointment soon became a full time one and I was able to move the Urology Department from the Whittington Hospital to the Royal Northern Hospital and all our elective surgery was performed there. A great many new innovations, including percutaneous renal surgery, were introduced and a book *Percutaneous Renal Surgery* by Wickham & Miller was published in 1986.

With help from the X-ray department, the new technique of sedoanalgesia, (sedation plus analgesia), revolutionised urological 'day case' surgery. A very strong academic input resulted in the production of three MD degrees and the publication of many research papers.

The success of the urological department at the Royal Northern Hospital can be related to the closure in 1986 of the accident and emergency department. In effect it became an elective hospital without emergency admissions. The beds could therefore be carefully controlled; and operating lists were managed very efficiently. It is interesting to draw a parallel with the modern day independent treatment centres which operate in the same way.

The second aspect of its surgical success was the focus on pelvic surgery. Professor Albert Singer's gynaecological unit developed a worldwide reputation in both laser surgery and research. Mr Russell Lock FRCS led the rectal surgical department. All aspects of pelvic surgery were covered and a very large number of major pelvic operations were able to take place between the three specialties.

The proximity of the ward immediately adjacent to the operating theatre meant a very rapid turnover. The experience of the nursing staff was second to none and Mary Gleason, theatre superintendent, ruled the operating theatres with a rod of iron. This ensured that there was never any 'down time', that is the time when an operating theatre suite was not in use; which is now seen so frequently. Dr Raja Jayaweera and Dr Pat Lee masterminded the anaesthetic services which allowed all these developments to take place.

Dr Jenny Dyson in the Pathology Department, provided an exemplary histology service in teaching the many post-graduate students who came to the Department.

Dr Geraint James' wonderful MRCP course was moved to the Whittington Hospital but the time slots were replaced by surgical teaching and the courses were run by the three surgical departments of the hospital.

Dr Gurcharan Rai, consultant in Care of

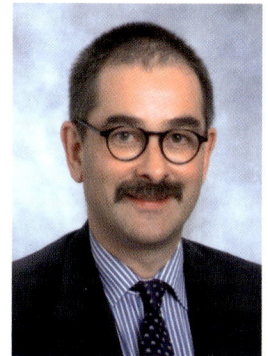

Mr Ronald Miller MS FRCS FRGS.

Photograph courtesy Mr Ronald Miller

the Elderly and Dr Roy Davies, cardiologist, were the physicians who closely supported our surgical unit and ensured the prompt discharge so essential for an efficient unit.

The Royal Northern Hospital had an unparalleled reputation with its patients, and despite its dilapidated buildings was much loved. The atmosphere was caring and efficient and the wards and corridors were spotlessly clean despite their age.

The hospital survived a major fire in its theatre block, which fortunately did not affect the oxygen storage or the whole department might have been blown up! The hospital was finally closed with services transferred to the Whittington Hospital. This was a sad day.

Professor Albert Singer PhD DPhil FRCOG. My years at the Royal Northern Hospital as consultant and Professor of Gynaecology (1981–1992)

I joined the staff of the Whittington & Royal Northern Hospitals in January 1981 having come from the position of Reader in Obstetrics and Gynaecology at the University of Sheffield.

I trained in Australia and obtained my basic medical and postgraduate degrees in Obstetrics and Gynaecology as well as a PhD at Sydney University before coming to Oxford on a Nuffield Dominion Travelling Fellowship in May of 1970 and obtained a DPhil from Oxford University in 1973.

My major interest has always been in carcinoma of the cervix and my PhD and DPhil were on aspects of the origins and the natural history of this disease, being one of the first to describe the possible linkage between the human papilloma virus and cervical neoplasia. I also established with Mr Joseph Jordan, (then a junior lecturer in gynaecology at Birmingham), the British Colposcopy Society in 1972; the forerunner of the British Society for Colposcopy and Cervical Cytology with currently over 2000 members.

My interest in colposcopy and in the management of cervical pre-malignancy developed in the University of Sheffield and I then brought this expertise to the Royal Northern Hospital in London. I was appointed in and commenced working there in January 1981. I immediately set about establishing a colposcopy clinic but was allowed no more than one four-hour clinic on a Friday morning. However within 10 years the service had grown to one of the largest in Europe with over 3,500 patients seen annually. Of these just over 2,000 patients were new referrals. The clinic established CO_2 laser therapy in 1984 which soon became adopted nationwide.

In mid 1981 the first colposcopy teaching course took place at the Whittington Hospital and this was the forerunner of eighty-seven such courses over the next twenty-six years. Most of the practising colposcopists within the United Kingdom have been to these courses, as have many from abroad. As well as these courses, twice yearly CO_2 laser treatment courses were run over five years from 1984-88 at the Royal Northern Hospital. Many of the leading European CO_2 laser laparoscopists and lower genital tract surgeons had their first experience at these courses. Professor Yona Tadir from Israel, one of the pioneers in laparoscopic therapy, taught on a number of these courses.

When the Royal Northern Hospital closed, the clinic moved to the Whittington Hospital to newly established premises partly financed by proceeds from the colposcopy training courses. Dr Jane Chomet a local general practitioner, and Dr Betty Mansell, a clinical assistant and then consultant, helped me re-establish colposcopy and lower genital tract clinics at the Whittington Hospital.

At the Royal Northern Hospital basic research was carried out in conjunction initially with Professor Denis McCance (from Guys Hospital) and then with Professor David Latchman, Dr Linda Ho, and Dr George Terry, eminent scientists in the field of molecular biology at University College, London. Some of the initial ground breaking studies on human papilloma virus originated from the team at the Royal Northern Hospital which included brilliant young researchers who in later years became heads of Professorial and National Health units.

Dr Michael Campion an enthusiastic Australian who worked with me over a two-year period during the 1980s was one of these researchers and helped publish some of the early work on the natural history of human papilloma virus in the male. Professor Sun Kuie Tay, now Professor at Singapore University, with Dr Campion and Dr Simon Barton, now consultant in genitourinary medicine at Chelsea and Westminster Hospital, published some of the initial studies on immune mechanisms operating in the cervix.

Some of the equipment used in the colposcopy clinic at the Royal Northern Hospital was funded by generous grants from the GHE Bequest which was an endowment charity established in the 1940s at the Royal Northern Hospital. Altogether some twenty-seven research fellows passed through the Royal

Northern Hospital during the years 1981–1990. The influence of the Royal Northern Hospital colposcopy and lower genital tract service on the British gynaecological scene was highly significant not only in its production of academic work but also in the innovative practical methods that its personnel pioneered and that subsequently became standard.

My years at the Royal Northern Hospital were a very fruitful period for research, both clinical and basic. The hospital had a unique reputation in the delivery of high quality clinical care. I endeavoured not only to continue this reputation with my colleagues but also to apply basic research findings to clinical practice. The ambience of the hospital, being as compact and functional as it was, with minimal bureaucratic managerial interference allowed this marriage of clinical and basic research to prosper. When the time came for closure I felt that a golden era in my professional life had ended.

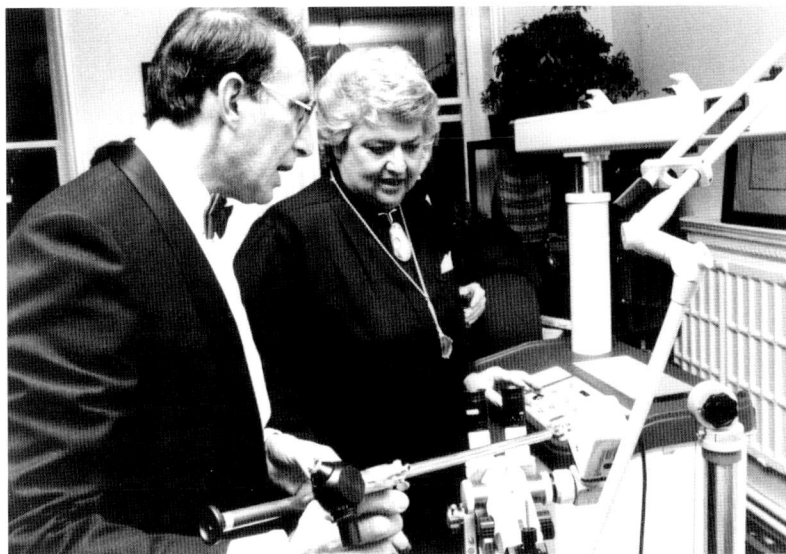

Professor Albert Singer is seen holding a laser laparoscope; also seen is a CO_2 laser machine and on the right is Claire Rayner. The event was at a celebratory dinner, 1985. Claire Rayner OBE, writer and broadcaster was also a former Gold Medallist in nursing at the Royal Northern Hospital School of Nursing, 1954.
Photograph 1985, courtesy Professor Albert Singer

The Honeywell Modular Operating Theatre systems

23

In the early 1960s the general design of the operating theatre systems in British hospitals had not changed much since the 1930s. About this time great development in surgical techniques were taking place. Open-heart surgery and hip-replacement were but two of pioneering procedures.

There was a growing realisation on the part of surgeons and theatre staff that if this type of surgery was to be successful, then the conditions prevailing needed to be improved. The greatest risk to success was, and still is, unexpected infections to the patient, often causing death or many years of pain.

Sterilisation techniques for instruments were of a reasonably good standard, but the environment in which they were used were not. Very few theatres boasted 'full' air conditioning, i.e. heating, cooling, humidification and filtration. Surgical staff were now being required to carry out operations lasting many hours with great discomfort to themselves and danger to patients and with open wounds exposed for long periods.

Though new hospitals were being planned and built, many centres of excellence in the surgical field were old Victorian hospitals where rebuilding and upgrading of facilities was almost impossible and of course, expensive.

The Modular Operating Theatre system

At this time a British company, New Electronic Products Limited, put together a design team with a view to producing a prefabricated operating theatre, which could be quickly assembled and installed in an existing building to provide an ultra clean, temperature and humidity-controlled environment for surgery. Very shortly after the formation of this team the company was taken over by Honeywell Controls Limited, a British subsidiary of Minneapolis Honeywell Inc. USA. Honeywell's strength, at that time, was in the field of environmental control systems.

The design parameters for this new product, named the Honeywell Modular Operating Theatre were: -

- All components should be factory manufactured to the highest possible standards of finish.

- The construction should be based on modular system, allowing operating theatres of different sizes to be provided according to space available and all types of surgery to be performed.

- All standard theatre equipment, operating lights, x-ray view screens, diathermy and other technical equipment should be supplied and fitted at the time of installation.

- It should be easily assembled on site, like a Meccano set.

- It must come complete with an integral air-conditioning plant and air filtration to a very high standard and be very easy to clean and maintain.

In about 1964, the first installation took place at Hammersmith Hospital, West London. The modular theatre was designed in conjunction with Professor Dennis Melrose, the pioneer cardiac physiologist at Hammersmith Hospital: surgeons and staff also provided enormous input to the design requirements.

In 1955, Professor Melrose helped Honeywell to design and construct the first United Kingdom heart-lung machine.

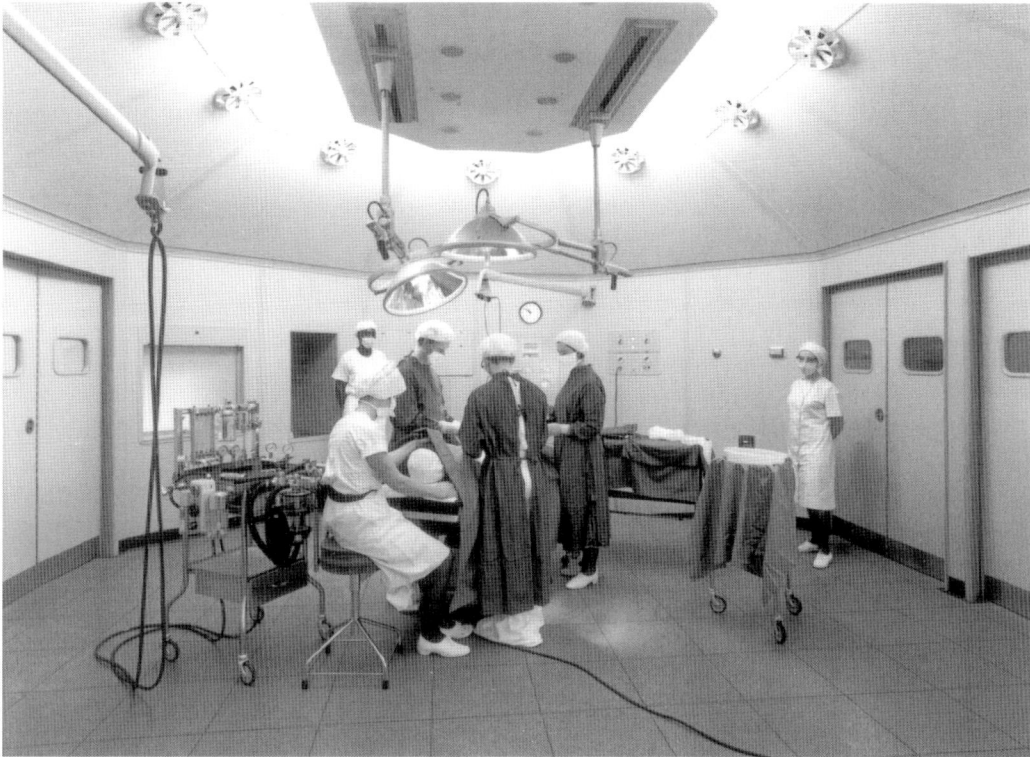

A Honeywell Operating Theatre, Royal Northern Hospital 1967.
Photography by Ronald Chapman FRPS.
Courtesy Corporation of London Metropolitan Archives.
Ref. H33/RN/PH/01/02

The prototype theatre was an immediate success, with infection rates and theatre staff tempers reduced considerably! As a result two more were installed there and were certainly in use for at least twenty years.

Over the next ten years, over one hundred units were built, including three at the Royal Northern Hospital, which were formally opened in 1967 by Sir Arthur Porritt KCVO MCh PRCS, Past President of the Royal College of Surgeons. Four Honeywell operating theatres were built for Moorfields Eye Hospital. It is interesting to note that the six Honeywell theatres installed at Clinique St Jean, Brussels, are still in use to this day. No doubt there are others

Technical information

The Honeywell Modular Operating Theatre is an octagonal construction with a sloping, tent-like roof. Conditioned air was supplied through ceiling diffusers incorporating five micron terminal filters. The air was vented out through self-sealing vents in the walls at low level. This ensured that a positive pressure was maintained within the theatre at all times, even when the doors were opened, only conditioned air could enter the room.

The fabric of the theatre consisted of self-supporting steel frames into which prefabricated wall and ceiling panels were fitted. The panels were comprised of melamine, aluminium sheet, plywood and foam insulation. This provided walls and ceilings that could be easily cleaned, electrically screened and thermally insulated; high quality conductive flooring was also fitted.

Each theatre included a 'clean' and a 'dirty' hatch mounted in the wall to provide a double door air-lock system for the supply of sterile instruments and disposal of used equipment and other waste. The whole system was engineered around the need to maintain the utmost cleanliness within the surgical environment.

Derek Bartlett, one time sales-manager,
Honeywell Medical Division UK,
kindly provided the above account

Nursing at the 'Northern' 1900s – 1970s

24

THE GREAT NORTHERN CENTRAL HOSPITAL, HOLLOWAY, LONDON
Royal Charter of Incorporation and Regulations 1911

Section 10 – The Matron

1. She shall; devote her whole time and attention to the affairs of the hospital and shall not be absent for a night without the permission of the House Committee.

2. She may suspend, at her discretion, any nurse for misconduct or inefficiency, until the next meeting of the Nursing Committee, to whom she shall report such suspension in writing.

3. The Matron shall provide for the due training of each probationer in every department of the hospital, including Medical and Surgical Wards, Operation Theatre, Surgery and Out-Patient Department. She shall hold classes at least once a week, except during the months of July, August and September for the teaching of practical nursing.

4. She shall visit all parts of the Hospital at least twice a week to see that they are clean and in proper order, and that Nurses and Female Servants are attentive to their duties. She shall preside at the Nurses' meals.

Section 11 – Nursing Staff

1. Any Sister, Nurse, or probationer may be suspended by the Matron for misconduct, neglect of duty, or inefficiency and such suspension shall be reported to the house Committee, who have powers of dismissal.

2. The Sisters, Nurses and Probationers are under the direction and control of the Matron, and they shall obey such general orders and instructions in regard to dress, hours of rest, recreation etc.

3. They shall not receive any fee, gratuity, or present of any kind from patients, friends of patients, or other persons, under any pretence whatever, on pain of dismissal.

4. They shall not be absent themselves from their duties, nor have any friends to visit them without the permission of the Matron.

Great Northern Central Hospital (Royal Northern Hospital), Holloway Road c.1900s

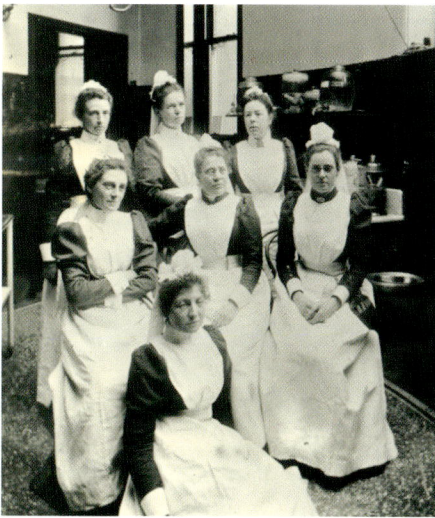

Group of nurses, early 1900s

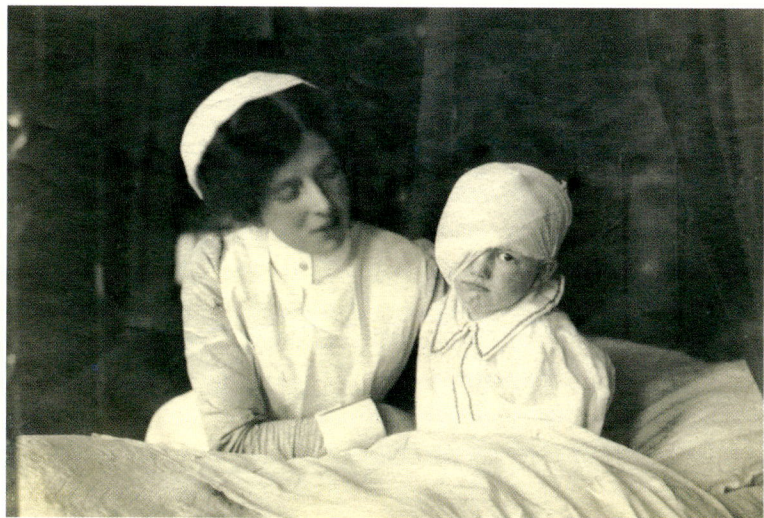

Possibly an eye-operation, post-operative c.1912

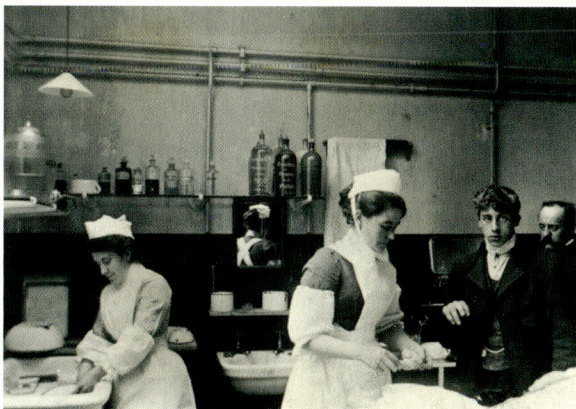

Nurses at work in the surgery c.1912

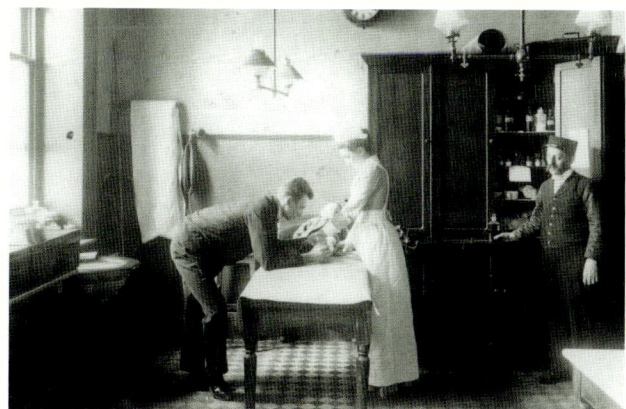

Nurse assisting a House Officer with the examination of a child c.1912

Images Courtesy Royal Northern Hospital Archives, Whittington Hospital

Preliminary Training School, Highbury Crescent c.1950s

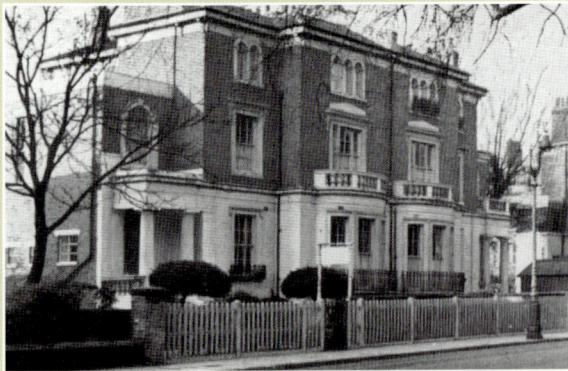

The Preliminary Training School, Highbury Crescent 1950s

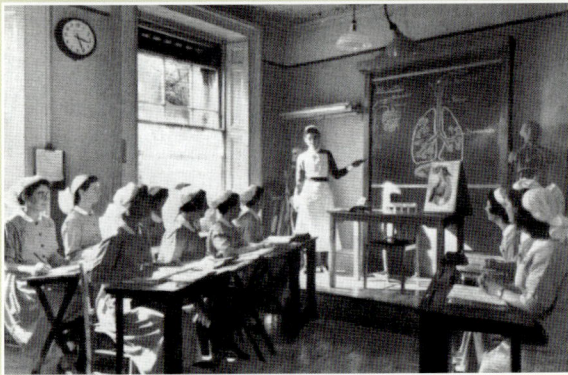

A lecture at the training school 1950s

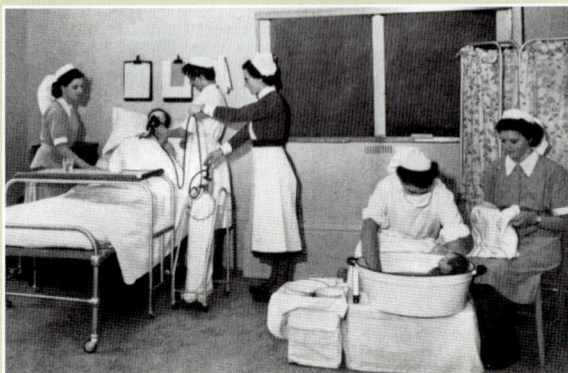

A practical class at the training school

Above images courtesy The Royal Northern Hospital 1856–1956', *Eric CO Jewesbury 1956*

The Preliminary Training School for Royal Northern Hospital Nurses was originally situated at Bryett Road near the hospital. Two adjacent houses, numbers eleven and twelve became available at Highbury Crescent, Islington. The houses were modernised and combined to form new Preliminary Training School, which was opened in 1952.

A Royal Northern Hospital League was formed in 1925 and Annual Reunions were held at the hospital. An annual Nurses Graduation Day in November was instituted in 1951 and in 1952, the Duchess of Gloucester came to present the nurses' prizes and toured the hospital.

In 1956, the Hospital nursing staff included 35 sisters, about 50 trained nurses and about 120 nurses in training.

Extract from The Royal Northern Hospital 1856–1956, *Eric CO Jewesbury 1956*

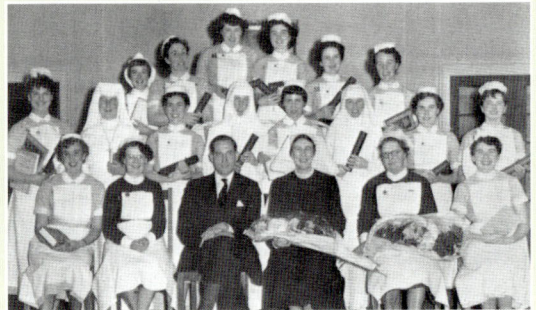

Nurses Graduation Day, November 1955. Including the Matron, Miss G.Darvill, the Hospital Group Secretary, Mr Frank Gray and two Sister Tutors

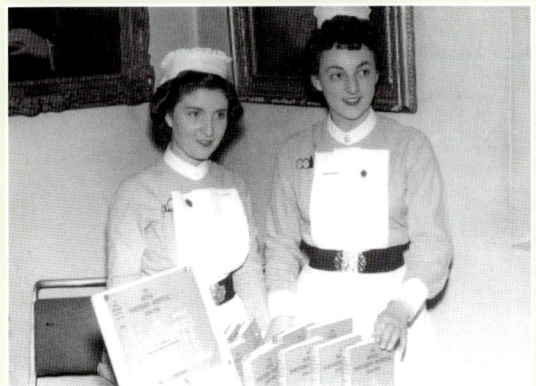

Staff Nurses displaying Dr Jewesbury's books for sale 1956 at the Royal Northern Hospital Centenary year

Courtesy Royal Northern Hospital Archives, Whittington Hospital

Royal Northern Hospital, Holloway Road c.1960s

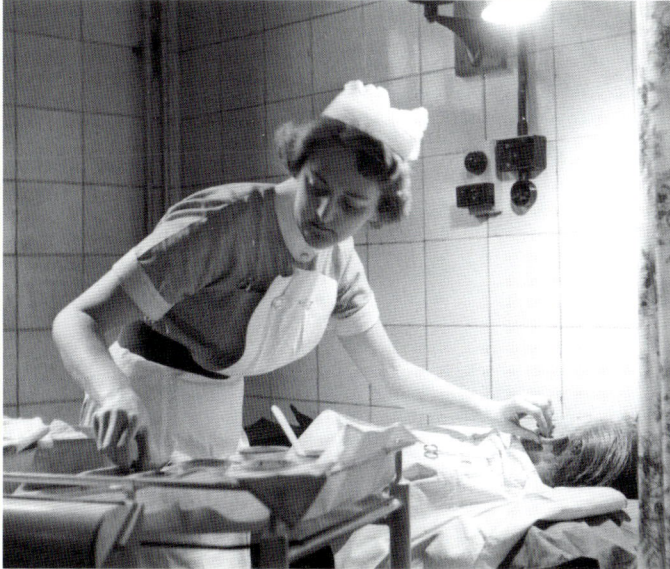

Nurse performing 'aural toilet'

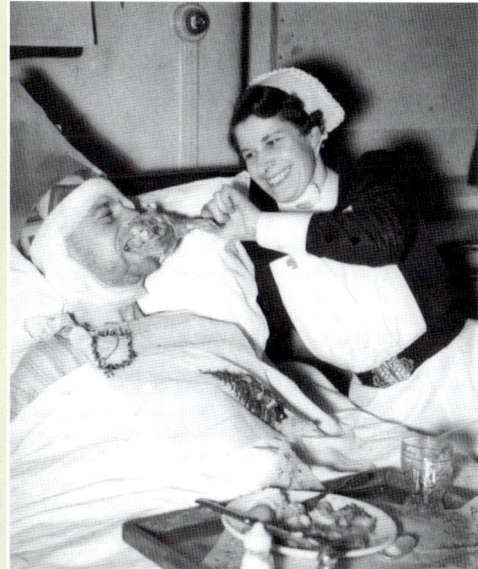

Sister giving a helping hand

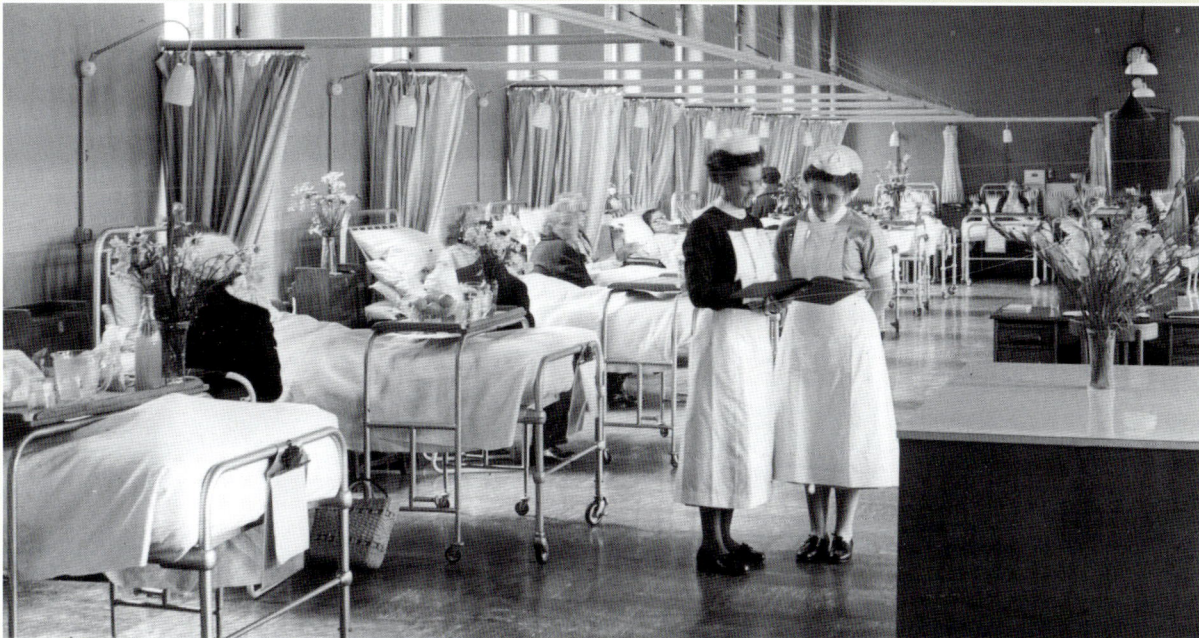

Sister in discussion with Staff Nurse

Images courtesy the Royal Northern Hospital Archives, Whittington Hospital

Royal Northern Hospital, Holloway Road c.1970s

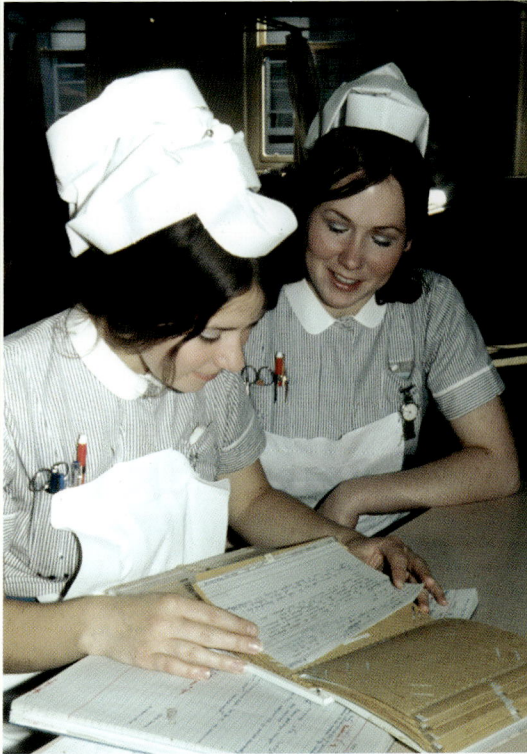

Nurses in discussion, possibly at a 'handover' period

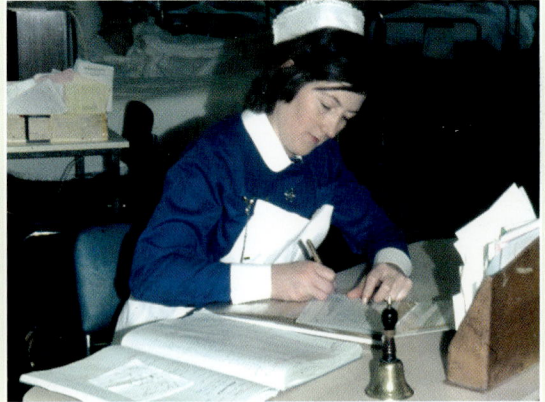

A quiet moment; Sister writing her report

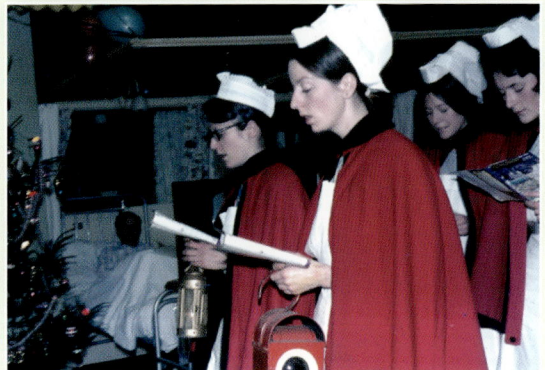

Traditional Christmas carols on the ward

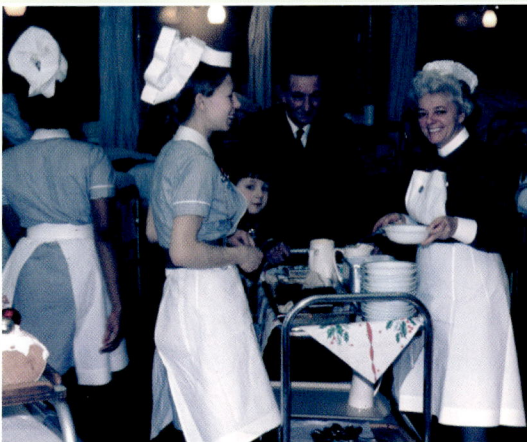

Sister serving Christmas fare

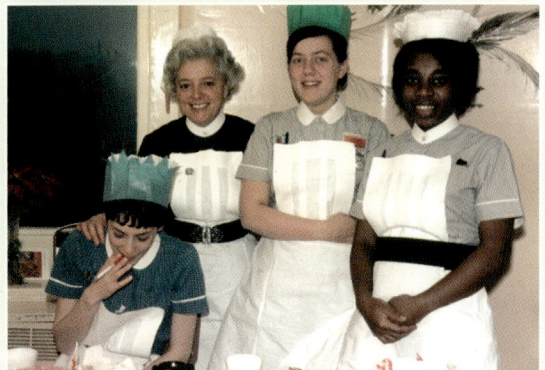

A happy moment!

Images courtesy Royal Northern Hospital Archives, Whittington Hospital

Closure of the Royal Northern Hospital – 1992

25

The old building of the Royal Northern Hospital including the façade, has been preserved, but total refurbishment has been carried out inside the building. The wrought iron staircase is probably all that remains of the interior of the original building. The other hospital buildings were completely demolished in 1992, which include the round wards, the out-patients department and St David's Wing.

The new building is named the Northern Health Centre, which houses community health services and a group general medical practice. A large number of flats have been built on the remaining site.

In 1923 the war memorial arch, designed by Percy Adams FRIBA, was built as part of a new Casualty Department of the Royal Northern Hospital. The memorial arch remains in Manor Gardens and behind the iron gates on

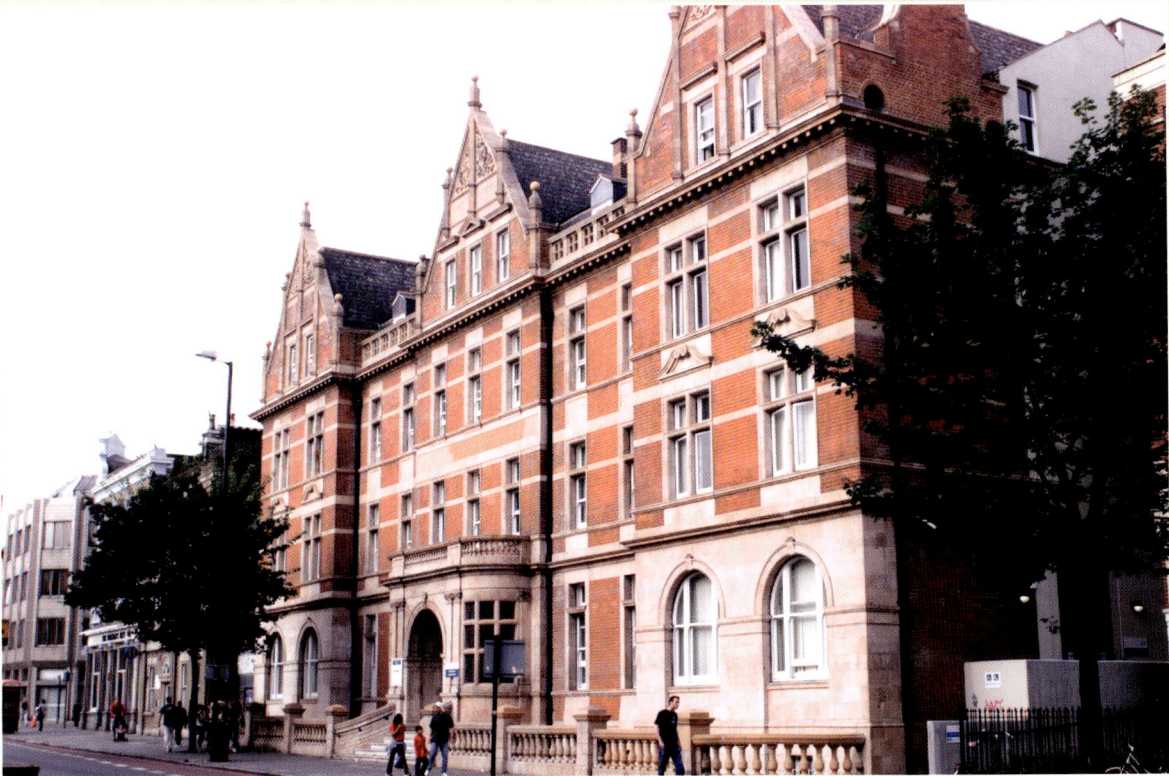

The Northern Health Centre 2002 (formerly the Royal Northern Hospital).
Courtesy Media Resources, University College London

either side of the archway, inscribed in Portland stone, there are walls bearing the names of the borough's 1,307 war dead. On each side is the inscription:

'TO THE MEMORY OF THOSE ISLINGTONIANS WHO MADE THE SUPREME SACRIFICE IN THE GREAT WAR 1914–1919'.

In July 1948 with the advent of the National Health Service, the Royal Northern Hospital ceased to be a voluntary hospital, and became a state hospital.

The Royal Northern Hospital finally closed its doors in 1992, thus ending one hundred and thirty six years (1856–1992) of continuous service to the people of Islington and beyond.

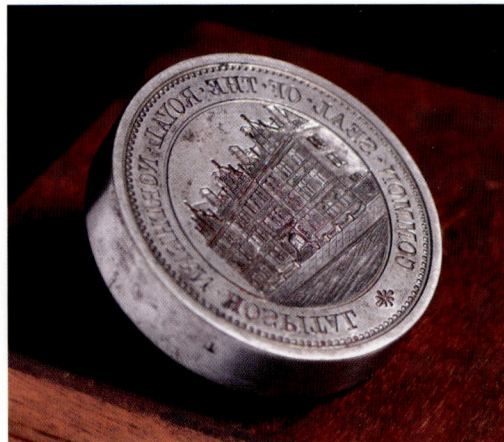

Hospital seal.
Courtesy Royal Northern Hospital Archive, Whittington Hospital

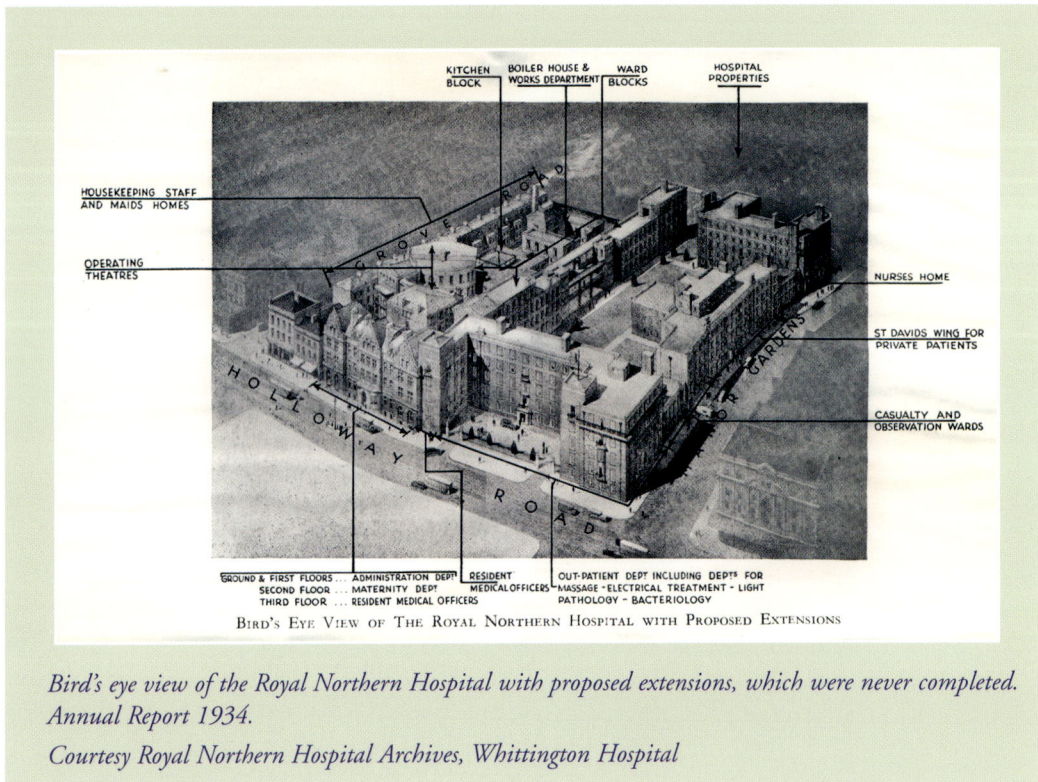

BIRD'S EYE VIEW OF THE ROYAL NORTHERN HOSPITAL WITH PROPOSED EXTENSIONS

Bird's eye view of the Royal Northern Hospital with proposed extensions, which were never completed. Annual Report 1934.

Courtesy Royal Northern Hospital Archives, Whittington Hospital

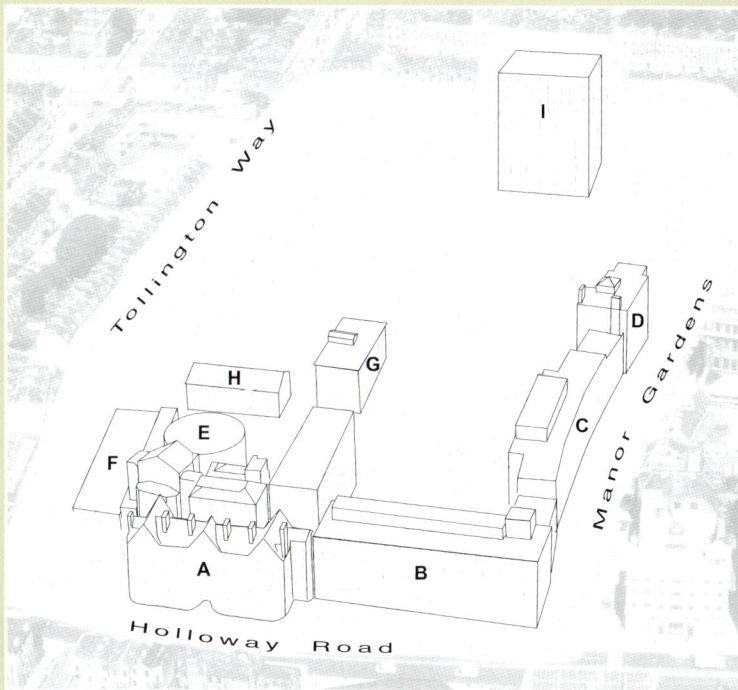

Key

A   Original old Royal Northern Hospital building

B   New Out-patient Department

C   St David's Wing for private patients

D   Old Nurses Home

E   Round Wards

F   Operating theatres (Honeywell theatres)

G   Beecham laboratory

H   Engineer's Department

I   Gloucester House (Nurses Home)

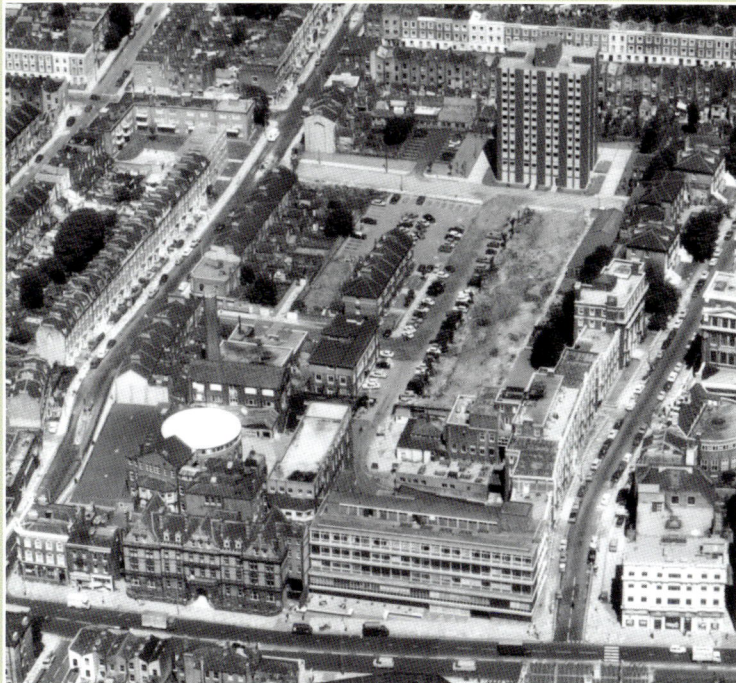

Aerial View of the Royal Northern Hospital in the 1970s.

Courtesy Royal Northern Hospital Archives, Whittington Hospital

Bibliography

General	© Fildes LV. *A Victorian Painter*. London: Michael Joseph 1968. © Graham H. *Eternal Eve*. William Heinemann 1950. © Humphries S V. *The Life of Hamilton Bailey*. Ravenswood Publications Ltd 1973. © Jewesbury ECO. *The Royal Northern Hospital 1856–1956*. H K.Lewis & Co Ltd. 1956. Marston A. *Hamilton Bailey A Surgeon's Life*. © London: Greenwich Medical Media Ltd. 1999. © Murley R. *Surgical Roots and Branches*. London: The British Medical Journal, 1990. © Sneader W. *Drug Discovery: The Evolution of Modern Medicines*. John Wiley & Sons Ltd 1985.
Chapter 1	Dee Cook, archivist, Society of Apothecaries of London, personal communication. Jewesbury ECO. *The Royal Northern Hospital 1856–1956*: 1, 2, 6–9. *The Great Northern Central Hospital, Holloway, London. Royal Charter of Incorporation and Regulations 3rd August 1911*: 3, 4. The Royal Northern Hospital Archives, Whittington Hospital.
Chapter 2	*The Lancet,* 13 November 1869.
Chapter 3	Banks MW. *British Medical Journal*. 8 October 1892: 787, 788. Dr Gustavus Murray, obituary. *Lancet*, 20 August 1887: 394. Rinsler Dr Albert. *The Journal of Medical Biography*. Vol 1: 3 August 1993. Reproduced with the permission of the Royal Society of Medicine Press, London. Rinsler Dr Albert. *The Doctor,* dissertation, DHMSA examination 1990. The Society of Apothecaries of London.
Chapter 4	Potter J. *Robert Bridges. (1844–1930)*. St Bartholomew's Hospital Journal, March 1954: 62–65. Robert Bridges, obituary. *St Bartholomew's Hospital Journal,* May 1930: 140. St Bartholomew's Hospital Archives.

Chapter 5	*Plarr's Lives of the Fellows.* Vol 1: 7 Royal College of Surgeons of England.
	Mr Ravi Kunzru MS FRCS DHMSA, personal communication.
Chapter 6	Jewesbury ECO. *The Royal Northern Hospital 1856–1956.* 53, 54, 63.
	An account of the Rise and Progress of the Great Northern Central Hospital 1856–1903. (Printed for private circulation ECB. Identity and date unknown). The Royal Northern Hospital Archives, Whittington Hospital.
Chapter 7	Photographic collection 1912. The Wellcome Library London.
Chapter 8	Jewesbury ECO. *The Royal Northern Hospital 1856–1956:* 97.
Chapter 9	*Royal Northern Group of Hospitals Annual Report 1932.* Royal Northern Hospital Archives, Whittington Hospital.
Chapter 10	Jewesbury ECO. *The Royal Northern Hospital 1856–1956:* 11–113.
	Royal Northern Group of Hospitals Annual Report 1931.
Chapter 11	*Royal Northern Group of Hospitals Annual Report 1937.* Royal Northern Hospital Archives, Whittington Hospital.
Chapter 12	Barrington-Ward Sir Lancelot KCVO ChM FRCS, autobiography. Unpublished manuscript 1953, courtesy Dr Breda Barrington-Ward.
	Plarr's Lives of the Fellows. Vol 4: 29 Royal College of Surgeons of England.
Chapter 13	Lord Horder GCVO DCL MD FRCP, obituary. *The British Medical Journal,* August 20 1955.
Chapter 14	Jonathan Evans, archivist, Royal London Hospital, personal communication.
	The London Hospital Gazette. Vol 21 December 1914. The Hamilton Bailey Archive, Royal London Hospital Archives.
	Plarr's Lives of the Fellows. Vol 4: 18 The Royal College of Surgeons of England.
Chapter 15	Robert McNeill Love MS FRCS. *Plarr's Lives of the Fellows.* Vol 6: 243 The Royal College of Surgeons of England.
Chapter 16	*Plarr's Lives of the Fellows.* Vol 250 The Royal College of Surgeons of England.
	Sir Reginald Murley Memorial Address. 11 December 1997. Sir Terence English KBE FRCP FRCS, personal communication.

Chapter 17	Panter G. *The Royal Northern Hospital in the 'Blitz'.* Royal Northern Hospital Publication (undated). *Royal Northern Group of Hospitals Annual Report 1940.* World War II. Imperial War Museum. Printed Books section, personal communication.
Chapter 18	Munk W. *The Role of the Royal College of Physicians of London.* Vol 2 London 1878. *Nursing Mirror,* 25 Jan 1941. The British Library. Panter G. *The Royal Northern Hospital in the 'Blitz'.* Royal Northern Hospital publication (undated). *Royal Northern Group of Hospitals Annual Report 1940.* Schuster N. *The Royal Chest Hospital. British Medical Journal,* 17 October 1953.
Chapter 19	Cannings RB. *City of London Maternity Hospital, City Road. A Short History 1922.* City of London Maternity Hospital publication. Cannings RB. *The City of London Maternity Hospital in the 'Blitz'.* The Medical Press and Circular, June 1943. Vol CCIX. Warner BJ (Beryl). *History of the City of London Maternity Hospital.* Northern Lights, quarterly staff magazine of the Northern Group of Hospitals. June 1955 No 4, September 1955 No 5.
Chapter 20	Dr W Alan Jennings PhD FInstP FIPEM, personal account.
Chapter 21	Dr Adrian Thomas FRCP FRCR, personal communication. Marion Frank OBE Hon DSc FCR, personal account.
Chapter 22	Personal accounts. Dr D Geraint James MD FRCP. Mr Ronald Miller MS FRCS FRGS. Professor Albert Singer PhD FRCOG. Sharma O. *A small United Nations – a memorable period.* *British Medical Journal.* Vol 319: 1468, 4 Dec 1999.
Chapter 23	Derek P Bartlett, personal account.
Chapter 24	*The Great Northern Central Hospital, Holloway, London. Royal Charter of Incorporation and Regulations.* 1911: 44, 46. Royal Northern Hospital Archives, Whittington Hospital.
Chapter 25	Planning Department London Borough of Islington, personal communication.